From Chocolate to Morphine

Also by Andrew Weil, M.D.

Also by Winifred Rosen

From Chocolate to Morphine

Everything You Need to Know
About Mind-Altering Drugs

Andrew Weil, M.D.
and Winifred Rosen

Revised Edition

HOUGHTON MIFFLIN COMPANY
BOSTON · NEW YORK

For information about permission to reproduce selections from
this book, write to Permissions, Houghton Mifflin Company,
215 Park Avenue South, New York, New York 10003.

Visit our Web site: www.houghtonmifflinbooks.com.

Library of Congress Cataloging-in-Publication Data
Weil, Andrew.
From chocolate to morphine : everything you need to know about
mind-altering drugs / Andrew Weil and Winifred Rosen. — Rev. ed.
p. cm.
Includes bibliographical references and index.
ISBN 0-618-48379-9 / 978-0-618-48379-2
1. Psychotropic drugs. I. Rosen, Winifred, 1943– II. Title.
RM315.W44 2004
615'.788—dc22   2004057677

Printed in the United States of America

Book design by Robert Overholtzer

DOC 10 9 8 7 6

The original title of this book was
Chocolate to Morphine: Understanding Mind-Active Drugs.

Contents

Acknowledgments

Honey Williams and Jeffrey Steingarten helped us in the early stages of our work, as did Woody Wickham and the late Dr. Norman Zinberg.

We are much indebted to Dr. Michael Aldrich and the Fitz Hugh Ludlow Memorial Library in San Francisco. Jeremy Bigwood provided good suggestions and needed infusions of energy. Special thanks go to the late Zig Schmitt for his company, support, and help in finding published source materials.

Leif Zerkin, editor of the *Journal of Psychoactive Drugs*, came up with recommendations for additional reading. Ken and Maria Robbins provided food and information. Dody Fugate of the University of Arizona gave us outstanding assistance.

Friends who helped us complete the manuscript include Richard Carey, Howard Kotler, Dr. David Smith, Sara Davidson, Helen Shewman, Dr. Tod Mikuriya, Jake Myers, Ethan Nadelmann, Jonathan Meader, Sue Fleishman, the late Tim Plowman, and Stanley and Jenine Moss.

We thank the late Dr. Richard Evans Schultes and the staff of the Harvard Botanical Museum for their help, and Anita McClellan, Karen Frankian, and Signe Warner for their part in tying together the many pieces of this work.

For the revised edition of 2004, we received much assistance from Lee Hunsucker and Stephanie Mayer and from the Drug Policy Alliance, especially from Ethan Nadelmann, Marsha Rosenbaum, and Jennifer Johnson-Spence. And we are greatly indebted to Polly Kummel, copy editor extraordinaire.

Authors' Note

MANY DRUGS MENTIONED in this book have three names: a chemical name that describes the molecule, a generic or common name, and a brand name owned by a company that markets the drug. For example, Valium is the brand name of a tranquilizer whose generic name is diazepam. The chemical name of this same drug is 7-chloro-l,3-dihydro-l-methyl-5-phenyl-2H-l,4-benzodi-azepin-2-one.

Because chemical names are long and cumbersome and useful only to chemists, we do not give them. We have tried to stick to generic names, which are printed in lowercase letters and followed, when relevant, by the most common brand names, enclosed in parentheses and capitalized. Thus: diazepam (Valium).

If the brand name is much better known than the generic name, as in the case of Valium, we will use it to refer to the drug after the first reference. Many "street" drugs, such as cocaine, LSD, and marijuana, do not have brand names.

WE HAVE SELECTED COMMENTS about mind-active drugs and accounts of experiences with them from users and nonusers of all ages. Short excerpts from many of these selections appear in the margins of the text. For fuller transcripts, see the appendix, beginning on page 223.

Preface to the 2004 Edition

IT IS NOW more than twenty years since this book first appeared, and we are sorry to say that it is as timely as ever.

Drugs pervade our society, abuse of them is rampant, and the authorities keep doing what they have always done, even though policies of eradicating drug plants, sealing borders, and zero tolerance for users have done nothing but made matters worse.

Over the years, we have received many letters from people telling us how much this book has helped them, from both those who read it as kids and those who read it as grownups and parents. Their responses reinforce the belief that led us to write *From Chocolate to Morphine* in the first place: truthful information about all drugs, presented clearly and nonjudgmentally, cannot cause harm.

We remain hopeful that truthful information will continue to do its work and that, as more individuals increase their knowledge of the real risks and benefits of mind-altering drugs, we will begin to see social change for the better.

We have updated the facts in these pages to reflect current realities. When we last revised the text, no one could have foreseen the epidemic of methamphetamine use in rural America or the popularity of Oxycontin, a medical opiate so favored in Appalachia that it has gained the nickname "hillbilly heroin." The bitter war over medical marijuana is also a recent phenomenon, pitting state and local governments and the will of the people against an implacable federal authority.

We hope that this new edition of *From Chocolate to Morphine* will provide a note of sanity in an otherwise irrational area of our cultural life.

February 2004

1. Straight Talk at the Start

D RUGS ARE HERE TO STAY.
History teaches that it is vain to hope that drugs will
ever disappear and that all efforts to eliminate them from
society are doomed to failure.

Throughout the twentieth century, Western society attempted
to deal with its drug problems through negative actions: by various wars on drug abuse implemented by repressive laws, disinfor-
mation, outrageous propaganda, and attacks on users, suppliers,
and sources of disapproved substances. These wars have been
consistently lost. More people are taking more drugs now than
ever before. Drug use has invaded all classes and ethnic groups
and has spread to younger and younger children. Also, more people *abuse* drugs now than ever before, and the drug laws are directly responsible for creating ugly and ever-widening criminal
networks that corrupt society and cause far worse damage than
the substances that they distribute.

The authors of this book were teen-agers and college students
in the 1960s. They had to confront the explosion of drug use of
that era and find out for themselves the benefits and dangers of
substances that they never learned about at home or in school.
One of us — Andrew Weil — has since become an expert on integrative medicine and optimum health. He has a medical degree
from Harvard and a rich background of travel among drug-using
cultures in other parts of the world, from the deserts of east Africa
to the jungles of South America. He draws on his training and his
professional and personal experience with most of the substances
described in these pages. As a recognized expert, he is frequently

invited to lecture on drugs to audiences of doctors as well as students, to testify on drugs in court trials, to write about them for textbooks and popular magazines, and to consult about them with government officials.

The other of us — Winifred Rosen — is a writer, the author of more than a dozen books for young people. The daughter of a psychoanalyst, she has long been interested in psychology and mental health. As a former high-school teacher and veteran of the 1960s, she has talked extensively about drugs with people of all ages and social backgrounds. She now does landscape gardening as well as writing.

We have been writing and traveling together on and off ever since we first met in San Francisco in 1968 (where we both served for a time as volunteers in the Haight-Ashbury Free Medical Clinic). Both of us believe that the present drug problem can change for the better only if society alters its strategy drastically. In this book we are not going to argue for or against drugs and will not side with either those who endorse them or those who oppose them. Instead, we will follow a middle course by presenting neutral information and will ask people on both sides to change some of their basic conceptions about drugs as a result of reading this material.

At the outset, we will insist that readers learn to distinguish drug use from drug abuse. As long as society continues to call all those who take disapproved substances "drug abusers," it will have an insoluble problem of enormous proportions. Real drug abusers are those in bad relationships with drugs (see Chapter 4), whether the drugs are approved or disapproved by society, and, unfortunately, little can be done to help these people, unless they want to change. Once people get into bad relationships with drugs, it is very hard to get them out. For most abusers, the only practical choice is total abstinence or continued abuse. (Some people may prefer that heroin addicts be in methadone treatment rather than on the street seeking heroin, but let us not kid ourselves: the "treatment" is just addiction to another narcotic.)

If society cannot do much about drug abuse once it develops, it certainly can, and should, work to *prevent* abuse. Instead of wasting so much time, money, and energy fighting the hopeless battle against existing drug abuse, society must begin to help people avoid becoming abusers in the first place.

Preventing drug abuse is a realistic goal. Two approaches are possible. One is to teach people, especially young people, how to satisfy their needs and desires without recourse to drugs. The second is to teach people how to form good relationships with drugs so that if they choose to use drugs, they will continue to be users and never become abusers.

The burden of this task will fall mainly upon parents and secondarily upon teachers; it is not a process that can be mandated by law or accomplished by public policy. However, laws and public policies must not undermine the work of parents and teachers by perpetuating irrational ideas about drugs, ideas rooted in fear and prejudice (see Chapter 2). The kind of instruction we would like to see will bear no resemblance to what is called "drug education" today. Drug education as it now exists is, at best, a thinly disguised attempt to scare young people away from disapproved drugs by greatly exaggerating the dangers of these substances. (The Drug Abuse Resistance Education [DARE] program is a perfect example.) More often than not, lectures, pamphlets, and video programs that take this approach stimulate curiosity, make the prohibited substances look more attractive to young audiences than they would be ordinarily, and make authorities appear ridiculous.

Parents and teachers will probably be open to efforts to interest children in alternatives to drugs. Adults will find it harder to support programs that teach young people how to form good relationships with drugs. With drugs so available and young people so disposed to experiment with them, good drug education is vital. The most that responsible adults can do is try to interest children in alternatives to drugs and give them information that will enable them to use drugs nonabusively should they choose to use them.

We have tried to make this book accessible to young people

by keeping our language and ideas simple and straightforward. When we were growing up, information like this was not available to the general public. As teen-agers, we struggled to get the facts, making many mistakes in the difficult process of learning the effects of drugs and adopting rules for living with them. We know how hard it is to grow up in a drug-filled world and hope our experience will be of use to younger generations.

To our teen-age readers we offer some general advice at the start:

You are growing up in a world awash in drugs. All of them can be used wisely or stupidly. Grownups will give you much misinformation about them and will often be dishonest or hypocritical about their own drug use (see Chapter 2). Many of your acquaintances will become involved with drugs, and you will have many opportunities to experiment with them yourself if you have not already done so. The fact that grownups exaggerate the dangers of drugs they disapprove of does not mean that those drugs have no dangers. *All drugs are dangerous.*

The only way you can be absolutely sure of avoiding problems with drugs is never to use them. That is a perfectly reasonable choice and may allow you more freedom than your drug-taking peers. Keep this in mind if you find yourself under pressure to take drugs. You may feel left out of certain groups if you abstain, but you will not really be missing anything. All of the experiences that people have with drugs can be had in other ways (see Chapter 13). If you do decide to experiment with drugs, whether approved or disapproved, make sure you know what the drugs are, where they come from, how they are likely to affect your body, and what precautions you should take to contain their potential for harm (see Chapters 6–11). Remember that forming good relationships with drugs is not easy, and maintaining good relationships takes work. Don't use drugs mindlessly and don't spend time around people who do.

If you are tempted to experiment with illegal drugs, keep in mind that being arrested can bring terrible consequences to you and your family. On the other hand, do not make the mistake of supposing that just because a drug is legal, it is safe. Some of the strongest and most dangerous drugs are legal.

You are less likely to encounter problems if you take dilute forms of natural drugs by mouth on occasion, especially if you take them for positive reasons that conform with rules that you have set for yourself (see Chapter 4). You are more likely to get into trouble if you take concentrated drugs frequently, particularly if you take them to escape feelings of unhappiness or boredom, or just because the drugs happen to be around.

It is a bad idea to take drugs in school. Even if school bores you, you have to be there, and mastering classroom skills is your ticket to freedom and independence in adult life. Drugs can interfere with your education by making it hard to pay attention, concentrate, and remember, or by involving you with people who reinforce negative attitudes about school.

Drugs are likely to be a source of friction between you and your parents. If your parents get upset with you for taking drugs, consider that they might have good reasons, such as valid fears about your safety, health, or psychological growth. Be willing to talk honestly with them and to hear their side with an open mind. Think about how you would feel in their place. What advice would you give your child if you found out he or she was taking drugs? Question your parents about the drugs that they use. Maybe they will agree to give up theirs if you will give up yours. Try to see what your experiences have in common with theirs. What alternatives to drug use can your parents suggest? If you can convince them that your drug use is responsible, you may be able to allay their anxiety. If their fears come from ignorance or misinformation, try to educate them, not by being emotional but by being well informed about the drugs you use. Give them this book to read as a background to your discussions of drug use.

Finally, remember that wanting to change your consciousness is not a symptom of mental illness or an unhealthy need to escape from reality. It is normal to want to vary your conscious experience (see Chapter 3). Drugs are just one way of doing it, though, and if you come to rely on them before you are grown up, you may not be able to appreciate a whole range of nondrug experiences that are more subtle but more rewarding over time. There is no question that drugs can get you high, but they are difficult to master and will fail you if you take them too often (see Chapter 13).

We hope that parents will read this book and use the information in it to help their children. We sympathize with parents. Odds are, you will have to confront the issue of a child's involvement with drugs. Before you react to the discovery that a son or daughter is using drugs, you should keep several points in mind:

A period of experimentation with drugs is today a normal phase of adolescence — a rite of passage that most children pass through unscathed.

Be sure that you have accurate information about the drugs that your child is using before you attempt to give advice. Children today are often well informed and contemptuous of antidrug information that they know to be false. Insisting that marijuana leads to heroin (see pages 142–43), or that ecstasy (MDMA) causes brain damage (see page 127), is a sure way to lose a child's attention and respect for your credibility about drug use.

Examine your own drug use before you question your child's. If your relationships with alcohol, tobacco, caffeine, and antianxiety drugs are not as good as they might be, a position against drug use may have little positive effect on your child. If you use illegal substances, your stand is further weakened by your own violation of drug laws.

It is important to create a climate of trust in which you and your child can communicate openly about difficult subjects like sex and drugs. Good communication is impossible when a parent assumes the role of detective, police officer, judge, or warden.

As we will stress throughout this book, a drug user is not necessarily a drug abuser. Meet your drug-using child with an open mind. Try to remember how you felt as a teen-ager. What forbidden activities did you engage in, and how easy was it for you to discuss them with your parents when you were discovered? Remember that, although the specific issues change from generation to generation, the basic conflicts and problems between adolescents and parents are universal and remarkably constant.

The primary responsibility for preventing drug abuse in your child is yours. Providing models of intelligent drug use is the best way to ensure that your child will use drugs rather than abuse them (if he or she uses them at all). It is well known that alcoholics tend to come from families where one or both parents are alcoholic, but it is less well known that alcoholics also tend to come from families where both parents are teetotalers. Apparently, the absence of a parental role model for successful drinking is the determining factor. The low incidence of alcoholism among Jews has long been ascribed to the integration of occasional social and ritual use of alcohol into Jewish family life. The more you encourage openness within your home and the better your own relationships are with the drugs you use, the more effective you will be at passing healthy drug attitudes and habits on to your child.

Make rules and set limits for your child about drugs. If your child respects you and the ways that you use alcohol, caffeine, and other substances, he or she will welcome guidelines. Be realistic about the rules you make. For example, if you feel strongly that you do not want illegal drugs in the house, you have the right to ban them. Of course, you must realize that your child may then use illegal substances outside the house.

Keep in mind that the main reason children experiment with drugs is to experience other states of consciousness (see Chapter 3). High states appeal to young people as much as they do to adults. Grown-ups enjoy racing cars and boats, hang-gliding, dancing, drinking, smoking, and many other consciousness-changing activities. Don't make your child feel that it is wrong to want these experiences. If you oppose the use of drugs to have such experiences, be prepared to forgo your own drug use. Also, be prepared to suggest alternatives. Alcohol is not an alternative. It is a drug, and the advantage of its legality is more than offset by its many dangers for users of any age (see pages 70–80).

Finally, consider the parallel problem of sexual experimentation, which, like drugs, is an adolescent rite of passage that parents have to deal with. Is it better to provide support for your child by expressing trust and offering reliable information about these issues or to force your child to seek information and experience without guidance and in risky ways? We believe the answer is obvious, in matters concerning sex and drugs alike.

Both of us have taught in schools and colleges and are aware that schools are now popular places for the distribution and consumption of drugs. We know that teachers are likely to be distressed by the prevalence of drug use among children today, especially when they encounter increasing numbers of students who cannot concentrate and have trouble learning because they are intoxicated on one substance or another.

Teachers have a special role in influencing children, but when they have to talk about heated, emotional subjects like drugs, teachers must bow to so many pressures that often they cannot follow their intuition or conscience. Teachers frequently must present drug education programs that are based on incorrect information and irrational attitudes. Acknowledging the falsity of the information may gain teachers the respect of students and allow the teachers to influence drug use for the better, but it may also cost them their jobs. We would like to see teachers inform themselves about drugs and work within the limits imposed on them to make classrooms places where young people feel free to discuss their interest in, experiences with, and conflicts about drugs.

As with successful sex education, to help students feel free to discuss drugs in class, teachers will have to clarify their own attitudes and be prepared to answer questions about their own uses and habits, since students will certainly ask. As in parental discussions of sex and drugs with teen-agers, honesty and consistency will give teachers credibility with their students. Given the political dimensions of the drug controversy, many teachers may just want to avoid the whole issue. We cannot blame them, since we know how vulnerable their positions are. Still, because teachers can contribute so much toward the prevention of drug abuse, we hope that they will try to find ways to change attitudes for the better.

Although we have written this book so that young people can read it, we intend it for doctors, lawmakers, members of the clergy, teachers, and users and nonusers, regardless of age. We have gathered this information from many sources, including our own experience, and, whenever possible, we have included first-person observations by others to create a more balanced overall picture. We have tried throughout to indicate how society can work to prevent drug abuse by encouraging the use of alternatives to drugs and encouraging the formation of good relationships with drugs when people choose to use them.

2. What Is a Drug?

MOST PEOPLE WOULD AGREE that heroin is a drug. It is a white powder that in tiny doses produces striking changes in the body and mind. But is sugar a drug? Sugar is also a white powder that strongly affects the body, and some experts say that it affects mental function and mood as well. Like heroin, sugar can be addicting. How about chocolate? Most people think of it as a food or flavor, but it contains a chemical related to caffeine, is a stimulant, and can also be addicting. Is salt a drug? Many people think that they cannot live without adding salt to their food, and it has dramatic effects on the body.

A common definition of the word *drug* is any substance that in small amounts produces significant changes in the body, mind, or both. This definition does not clearly distinguish drugs from some foods. The difference between a drug and a poison is also unclear. All drugs become poisons in high enough doses, and some poisons are useful drugs in low enough doses. Is alcohol a food, a drug, or a poison? The body can burn it as a fuel, just like sugar or starch, but it causes intoxication and can kill in overdose. Many people who drink alcohol crusade against drug abuse, never acknowledging that they themselves are involved with a powerful drug. In the same way, many cigarette addicts have no idea that tobacco is a strong drug, and many people who depend on coffee do not realize that they are addicted to a stimulant.

The decision to call some substances drugs and others not is often arbitrary. In the case of medical drugs — aspirin and penicillin, for example, which are used only to treat and prevent physical illness — the distinction may be easier to make. But talking about psychoactive drugs — substances that affect mood, perception, and thought — is tricky.

In the first place, foods, drugs, and poisons are not clear-cut categories. Second, people have strong emotional reactions to them. Food is good. Poison is bad. Drugs may be good or bad, and whether they are seen as good or bad depends on who is looking at them. Many people agree that drugs are good when doctors give them to patients in order to make them better. Some religious groups, such as Christian Scientists, do not share that view, however. They believe that God intends us to deal with illness without drugs.

When people take psychoactive drugs on their own, in order to change their mood or feel pleasure, the question of good or bad gets even thornier. The whole subject of pleasure triggers intense controversy. Should pleasure come as a reward for work or suffering? Should people feel guilty if they experience pleasure without earning it or suffering for it in some way? Should work itself be unpleasant? These questions are very important to us, but they do not have easy answers. Different people and different cultures answer them in different ways.

Drug use is universal. Every human culture in every age of history has used one or more psychoactive drugs. (The one exception is some Inuit, who were unable to grow drug plants in the Alaskan tundra and had to wait for white men to bring them alcohol.) In fact, drug-taking is so common that it seems to be a basic human activity. All societies, therefore, must come to terms with people's fascination with drugs. Usually, the use of certain drugs is approved and integrated into the life of a tribe, community, or nation, sometimes in formal rituals and ceremonies. The approval of some drugs for some purposes usually goes hand in hand with the disapproval of other drugs for other purposes. For example, some early Muslim sects encouraged the use of coffee in religious rites but had strict prohibitions against alcohol. On the other hand, when coffee came to Europe in the seventeenth century, the Roman Catholic Church opposed it as an evil drug but continued to regard wine as a traditional sacrament.

Everybody is willing to call certain drugs bad, but there is little agreement from one culture to the next as to which these are. In our own society, all nonmedical drugs other than alcohol, tobacco, and caffeine are viewed with suspicion by the majority. There are subgroups within our society, however, that hold very different opinions. Many North American Indians who use peyote and tobacco in religious rituals consider alcohol a curse. The most fervent members of the counterculture that arose in the 1960s regard marijuana and psychedelics as beneficial while rejecting not only alcohol, tobacco, and coffee but most other legal and illegal drugs as well. Classic heroin addicts — junkies — may reject psychedelics and marijuana as dangerous but think of narcotics as desirable and necessary. Some yogis in India use marijuana ritually but teach that opiates and alcohol are harmful. Muslims may tolerate the use of opium, marijuana, and qat (a strongly stimulating leaf) but are very strict in their exclusion of alcohol.

Furthermore, attitudes about which drugs are good or bad tend to change over time within a given culture. When tobacco first came to Europe from the New World, it provoked such strong opposition that authorities in some countries tried to stamp it out by imposing the death penalty for users. But within a century, its use was accepted and even encouraged by governments eager to exploit its revenue-earning potential. In the past century, Americans' attitudes toward alcohol shifted from nonchalant tolerance to antagonism strong enough to result in national prohibition and back to near-universal acceptance. And the debate over marijuana in the 1960s was mostly a conflict between an older generation that viewed the drug as evil and a younger generation that found it preferable to alcohol.

Students of behavior tell us that dividing the world into good and evil is a fundamental human need. The existence of evil provokes fear and demands explanation. Why is there sickness? Why is there death? Why do crops fail? Why is there war? And, most important, how should we act to contain evil and avoid disaster? One approach to resolving these questions attributes evil to external things and then prohibits, avoids, or tries to destroy those things. This is the process that gives rise to taboos.

Taboos tend to crystallize around those activities and substances that are most important to us. Food, sex, and pleasure are very important, and many taboos surround them — although, again, there is little agreement from culture to culture as to the particulars. Muslims and many Jews eat beef but not pork; some groups in India eat pork but not beef. Homosexuality is taboo in most modern Western cultures but has been fully accepted in the past and is still accepted today in certain parts of the world.

People who adhere to taboos justify them with logical reasons. Jews who do not eat pork like to think that this is because pigs are unclean and carried disease in times past. Many Christians argue that homosexuality is a sin because it perverts God's intended use of sex for procreation. Actually, the reasons for taboos are secondary; the basic process is the dividing of important things into good and evil — a form of magical thinking that tries to gain control over sources of fear. The reasons and justifications come later.

Because psychoactive drugs can give pleasure and can change the ways that people think, perceive the world, behave, and relate to each other, they invite magical thinking and taboos. When you hear arguments on the merits or dangers of drugs, even by scientific experts, remember that these may be secondary justifications of preexisting views that are deep-seated and rooted in emotion. (It is always easy for both sides to produce statistics and "scientific evidence" to support their position.)

Because people have many fears and desires about drugs, finding neutral information about them is difficult. In this book, we try to give unbiased facts about all the psychoactive drugs that people are likely to encounter today. We cannot say that we have no biases about drugs, but we think that we know what our biases are. Our strongest conviction is that drugs themselves are neither good nor bad; rather, they are powerful substances that can be put to good or bad uses. We are concerned with the relationships that people form with drugs, whether legal or illegal, approved or unapproved. We believe that by presenting neutral information about these substances, we can help people, especially young people, come to terms with drugs. Our purpose is not to encourage or discourage the use of any drug but rather to help people learn to live in a world where drugs exist and not get hurt by them.

SUGGESTED READING

The best book on the subject of how societies classify drugs as good and evil is *Ceremonial Chemistry: The Ritual Persecution of Drugs, Addicts, and Pushers* by Thomas Szasz (New York: Doubleday/Anchor, 1975). Szasz is a psychiatrist interested in the assumptions that lead people to call some kinds of behavior sick or wrong. His discussion of drugs and drug users as scapegoats is excellent.

A good general book on psychoactive drugs is *Uppers, Downers, All Arounders: Physical and Mental Effects of Drugs of Abuse* by Darryl S. Inaba and William E. Cohen (Ashland, Oreg.: Cris Productions, 1997). See also *Drugs of Abuse: An Introduction to Their Actions & Potential Hazards* (2004 edition, catalog #203) by Samuel Irwin, distributed by the Do It Now Foundation (www.doitnow .org/pages/203/toc.html) (last accessed April 2004).

A book written for junior-high and high-school students that gives a good overview of the subject is *Mind Drugs*, edited by Margaret O. Hyde (third edition; Brookfield, Conn.: Millbrook, 1998).

3. Why People Use Drugs

DRUGS ARE FASCINATING because they can change our awareness. The basic reason that people take drugs is to experience states other than normal, waking consciousness. Of course, there are many other ways to alter consciousness, such as singing, dancing, eating, fasting, falling in love, laughing, traveling, meditating, playing ball, going to concerts, movies, museums, and plays, mountain climbing, deep sea diving, reading, writing, and fantasizing. The list is probably endless, because it includes nearly all the activities that people put most of their time, energy, and hard-earned money into, suggesting that changing consciousness is something that people like to do.

Human beings appear to have an inborn need for periodic variations in consciousness. The behavior of young children supports this idea. Infants rock themselves into blissful states; many children discover that whirling, or spinning, is a powerful technique for changing their awareness; some also experiment with hyperventilation (rapid, deep breathing) followed by mutual chest squeezing or choking, and tickling to produce paralyzing laughter. Even though these practices may produce some uncomfortable results, such as dizziness or nausea, the whole experience is so reinforcing that children do it again and again, often despite parental objections. Since children all over the world engage in these activities, the desire to change consciousness does not seem to be a product of a particular culture but rather to arise from something basically human. As children grow older, they find that certain available substances put them in similar states. Drugs are attractive because they provide an easy, quick route to these experiences.

Humans have been seeking out and experimenting with psychoactive substances since the dawn of time. The impulse to find and ingest drug plants goes so far back and is so universal that it seems to be intrinsic to human nature and integral to the evolution of human culture.

Many drug users talk about getting high. Highs are states of consciousness marked by feelings of euphoria, lightness, self-transcendence, concentration, and energy. People who never take drugs also seek out highs. In fact, having high experiences from time to time may be necessary to our physical and mental health, just as laughing, interacting with others, and dreaming during sleep seem to be vital to our well-being. Perhaps that is why a desire to alter our normal consciousness exists in everyone and why people pursue the experiences even though there are sometimes uncomfortable side effects.

Although the desire to experience high states is at the root of all drug-taking, on a practical level people take drugs for a wide variety of reasons. These include:

Reinforcing religious practices. Throughout history, people have used drug-induced states to transcend their sense of separateness and feel more at one with God, nature, and the supernatural. Marijuana was used for this purpose in ancient India, and many psychedelic plants are still so used today by indigenous peoples in both North and South America. Alcohol has been used for religious purposes in many parts of the world; the role of wine in Roman Catholic and Judaic rites persists as an example. Among tribal cultures, psychoactive plants are often considered sacred — gifts from gods and spirits to unite people with the higher realms.

Expanding awareness and exploring the self. Curious individuals throughout history have taken psychoactive substances to explore and investigate parts of their own minds that are not ordinarily accessible. One of the most famous modern examples was the British writer and philosopher Aldous Huxley, who experimented extensively with mescaline in the 1950s. His book *The Doors of Perception* is a record of his investigations. The title comes from a line of William Blake's: "If the doors of perception were cleansed, every thing would appear to man as it is — infinite." Some other well-known "explorers" are Oliver Wendell Holmes, the nineteenth-century American physician, poet, and author, who experimented with ether; William James, the Harvard psychologist and philosopher of the late nineteenth century, who used nitrous oxide; Sigmund Freud, the father of psychoanalysis, who took cocaine; William S. Burroughs, a modern American novelist and user of opiates and many other substances; Richard Alpert (Ram Dass), a psychologist and guru, who has extensive experience with LSD and other psychedelics; and John Lilly, a medical researcher and philosopher, who experimented with ketamine. Many others who have followed this path have done so privately, keeping their experiences to themselves or sharing them only with intimate companions.

Treating disease. Because psychoactive drugs really make people feel different, doctors and patients have always relied heavily on them for dealing with the symptoms of illness. Opium, morphine, and alcohol were mainstays of nineteenth-century medicine, used to treat everything from menstrual cramps to epilepsy. (One eminent physician of the day proclaimed morphine to be "God's own medicine.") Tincture of marijuana was also a popular remedy. At the end of the nineteenth century, cocaine was promoted as a miracle drug and cure-all, and coca wine was the most widely prescribed drug for a time. Until recently, diazepam (Valium) held that distinction. This kind of treatment may work by distracting a patient's attention from symptoms and shifting it instead toward the good feeling of a high. Sometimes the medical problem will then go away on its own. Often, however, if there is no treatment of the underlying cause of the symptoms, the problem will persist, and the patient may go on to use the drug again and again until dependence results.

Altering moods. Many people take drugs to relieve anxiety, depression, lethargy, or insomnia or just because they feel bored. The view that unwanted moods are disease states that are treatable by taking medicines has now become widespread in our society. The chief proponent and greatest beneficiary of this way of thinking is the pharmaceutical industry, with the result that a great many of the legal medical drugs sold today are aimed at changing undesired moods. Young people not only see their parents using drugs in this way but also are influenced by advertisements and commercials that directly promote such behavior. Many people of all ages use nonmedical drugs, both legal and illegal ones, in this fashion.

Escaping tedium and despair. In the words of Aldous Huxley, "Most men and women lead lives at the worst so painful, at the best so monotonous, poor, and limited that the urge to escape, the longing to transcend themselves, if only for a few moments, is and has always been one of the principal appetites of the soul."

Facilitating and enhancing social interaction. Like sharing food, the ritual of taking drugs together is an excuse for intimacy; coffee breaks and cocktail ("happy") hours are examples of the way that approved drugs are used for this purpose. Disapproved drugs may draw people together even more strongly by establishing a bond of common defiance of authority. At the big rock concerts and Vietnam War protests of the 1960s, strangers often became instant comrades simply by passing a joint back and forth.

In different cultures, other drugs perform the same function. For example, South American Indians take coca breaks together, much as we take coffee breaks, and chewing coca leaves with a friend establishes an important social bond. For South Sea Islanders, drinking kava in groups at night is the equivalent of an American cocktail party.

In addition to the ritual significance with which drugs are invested, their pharmacological effects may also make social interac-

tion easier. Because alcohol lowers inhibitions, businesspeople often have drinks at lunch to encourage openness and congeniality.
Similarly, people on dates often drink to reduce anxiety and feelings of awkwardness. By producing alertness and euphoria, stimulants such as cocaine promote easy conversation, even among
strangers.

So important is this function of psychoactive drugs that many
people would find it difficult to relate to others if deprived of them.

Enhancing sensory experience and pleasure.   Human beings are
pleasure-seeking animals who are very inventive when it comes to
finding ways to excite their senses and gratify their appetites. One
of the characteristics of sensory pleasure is that it becomes dulled
with repetition, and there are only so many ways of achieving pleasure. As much time, thought, and energy have gone into sex as
into any human activity, but the possibilities of sexual positions
and techniques are limited. By making people feel different, psychoactive drugs can make familiar experiences new and interesting again. The use of drugs in combination with sex is as old as
the hills, as is drug use with such activities as dancing, eating, and
listening to or playing music. Drinking wine with meals is an example of this behavior that dates to prehistory and is still encouraged by society. There are those who say that a good cigar and a
glass of brandy make a fine meal complete. Pot lovers say that
turning on is the perfect way for a fine meal to begin. Psychedelic
drugs, especially, are intensifiers of experience and can make a
sunset more fascinating than a movie. (Of course, psychedelics
can also turn an unpleasant situation into a living nightmare.) Because drugs can, temporarily at least, make the ordinary extraordinary, many people seek them out and consume them in an effort
to get more enjoyment out of life.

Stimulating creativity.   Writers have traditionally used psychoactive substances as sources of inspiration. The English poet Coleridge's famous visionary poem, "Kubla Khan," was a transcription

> In Xanadu did Kubla Khan
> A stately pleasure dome decree:
> Where Alph, the sacred river, ran
> Through caverns measureless to man
> Down to a sunless sea.
>
> — opening lines of "Kubla Khan" (1798), by Samuel Taylor Coleridge
>   (1772–1834)

of one of his opium dreams. The French poet Charles Baudelaire took hashish as well as opium for creative inspiration. His compatriot, the novelist Alexandre Dumas, joined him in experiments with hashish. The American writer Edgar Allan Poe used opiates; some of the weirdness of his tales probably derives from his drug experiences. Sigmund Freud's early writings were inspired by cocaine; for a time, he actively promoted cocaine as a miracle drug. Innumerable novelists, poets, playwrights, and journalists have found their inspiration in alcohol. Many have paid the high price of becoming alcoholics.

Some traditional peoples turn psychedelic visions into art. In Mexico, for example, the Huichol Indians turn their peyote visions into yarn paintings. Other artists use other psychoactive drugs to help translate their visions into art. Diego Rivera, the best-known Mexican artist of the twentieth century, favored marijuana. The famous American abstract painter Jackson Pollock was a prodigious drinker and an alcoholic; he died at age forty-four in a car crash, the result of driving while intoxicated.

Among the earliest and most enthusiastic users of marijuana when it first surfaced in the United States in the 1920s were blues and jazz musicians, and musicians have been in the vanguard of the drug movement ever since. Some of the greatest jazz musicians were heroin addicts; countless others drank to excess. But nowhere are drugs consumed so conspicuously as in the world of rock music. Jimi Hendrix, Janis Joplin, Jim Morrison, Brian Jones, and Sid Vicious are just a few of the rock stars who died of drug overdoses at a young age. Elvis Presley overdosed at forty-two. Many other great artists, including Eric Clapton, Willy Nelson, James Taylor, and Johnny Cash, came perilously close to burning out on cocaine, narcotics, or alcohol before cleaning up their acts.

Improving physical performance.   Various drugs can enable people to perform out-of-the-ordinary feats. In the ancient Inca empire of Peru, relay runners used coca in order to be able to cover vast distances in the high Andes, carrying news and messages to all parts of the kingdom. Warriors throughout history have fortified themselves with alcohol before going into battle, to boost their courage and decrease sensitivity to pain. Many professional athletes today follow in this tradition, although drug testing has curtailed their uses of illegal stimulants. Baseball players still chew tobacco. Truckers still drive long distances on little sleep and a lot of methamphetamine.

Rebellion.   Because drugs are surrounded by powerful taboos, they are ideal vehicles for rebellious behavior. Breaking taboos is an obvious way to challenge the values of the "establishment." Children quickly learn that they can upset parents, teachers, doctors, and other authorities by taking forbidden substances. Adoles-

> You get into heroin because you have a lot of money in your pocket, and you can't go to video games all the time, and you think life is very trivial and very boring, and you look for other people who think the same.
>
> — seventeen-year-old woman, heroin addict

> I started shooting heroin at the age of twelve and was a
> junkie till I was fifteen. I went cold turkey eight or nine
> times, but after each cold turkey I'd see my old friends
> again, and then I'd go back to heroin.
>
> — nineteen-year-old woman, former heroin addict

cence typically entails the assertion of independence, often by
rejecting parental values. It is not surprising that adolescents frequently experiment with drugs. Unfortunately, the attempt to control drug-taking by making some substances illegal plays right
into the hands of rebellious children. And, of course, some adults
who have not outgrown adolescent traits continue to express re-
belliousness in the ways that they take drugs.

Going along with the crowd. Individuals who would not seek out
drugs on their own will often take them in a group, because not to
do so would be uncool. Although teen-agers may dislike the effects at first, they often take up smoking tobacco or marijuana in
order to fit in and be accepted, much as they might adopt a trendy
fashion style that does not suit them.

Using drugs because everyone else is using them is not a good
reason, but it is a very common one.

Establishing an identity and getting attention. Individuals or
groups may take up the use of a prohibited substance or abuse a
permitted one in order to define and advertise their specialness.
Adopting unusual or extreme drug styles may not be wise, but it
can be an effective way to get attention and recognition.

People's reasons for taking drugs are so varied that it's sometimes
hard to know what is motivating a person to take a particular drug
at any given time or why a person would choose to take one drug

rather than another. People take different drugs for different reasons at different times. And some people take drugs for no reason, purely out of habit.

SUGGESTED READING

Andrew Weil's *The Natural Mind: A Revolutionary Approach to the Drug Problem* (revised edition; Boston: Houghton Mifflin, 2004) examines drug-taking as a method of changing consciousness and speculates on why altered states of consciousness are important to us.

Society and Drugs by Richard H. Blum et al. (San Francisco: Jossey-Bass, 1970) is a good survey of drug use in various cultures throughout history. In *The Joyous Cosmology: Adventures in the Chemistry of Consciousness* (New York: Vintage, 1965), philosopher Alan Watts gives a colorful picture of states of consciousness induced by hallucinogenic drugs. Watts experimented with these substances as an explorer of the mind and a searcher for religious experience.

Shaman Woman, Mainline Lady: Women's Writings on the Drug Experience, edited by Cynthia Palmer and Michael Horowitz (New York: William Morrow, 1982), is an anthology covering many times and cultures. It gives a broad overview of different ways of using many drugs.

For an account of the healing power of laughter, see *Anatomy of an Illness* by Norman Cousins (New York: Bantam, 1991).

High Culture: Reflections on Addiction and Modernity, edited by Anna Alexander and Mark S. Roberts (Albany: State University of New York Press, 2003), addresses the prevalence of addiction in literature, philosophy, modern art, and psychology, including its effects on many prominent thinkers and writers.

The American Drug Scene: An Anthology, edited by James A. Inciardi and Karen McElrath (third edition; Los Angeles: Roxbury, 2000), is a collection of both contemporary and classic essays and articles on the changing patterns, problems, perspectives, and policies of both legal and illegal drug use.

A good overall textbook about drugs is *Drugs, Society, and Human Behavior* by Oakley Stern Ray and Charles J. Ksir (eighth edition; Boston: WCB/McGraw Hill, 1999).

4. Relationships with Drugs

THE DESIRE TO CALL some drugs good and others bad has given rise to the term *drugs of abuse*. Government officials and medical doctors frequently talk about drugs of abuse, by which they usually mean all illegal substances. In their view, anyone using these drugs is automatically guilty of drug abuse.

But what is drug abuse? To say that it is the use of a drug of abuse is circular and meaningless. We think that the use of *any* drug becomes abusive when it threatens a person's health or impairs one's social or economic functioning. People with respiratory disease who persist in smoking cigarettes are clearly abusing tobacco. Students who are booted out of class because they are too stoned to concentrate are abusing marijuana. Drinkers too drunk to hold down jobs are abusers of alcohol. Addicts who squander all their money on heroin, thereby impoverishing their families, are abusers of that drug. On the other hand, any drug can be used in a nonabusive fashion, even if it is illegal or disapproved. There are many people who consume tobacco, marijuana, alcohol, and heroin without abusing them, that is, they remain healthy and fulfill their social and economic obligations. Drug abuse is not simply a matter of what drug a person chooses to consume; rather, it depends on the relationship that an individual forms with that drug.

Many factors determine relationships with drugs. Obviously, the drug itself is one important factor; there is a whole science, pharmacology, devoted to finding out what drugs do.

Unfortunately, the effects of drugs are difficult to specify. Different people show different responses to the same dose of the same drug, probably because people differ in their biochemistry, just as they do in appearance. Even the same person may respond differently to the same dose of the same drug at different times. Pharmacologists attempt to minimize these variations by giving drugs to animals and people under controlled laboratory conditions. The results of these experiments enable pharmacologists to classify drugs into different categories. For example, they can show most psychoactive drugs to be either stimulants or depressants of the nervous system.

Laboratory experiments also show that the dose of a drug is a crucial variable. High doses of a substance may produce very different effects from low doses. Moderate doses of alcohol will make many people feel relaxed and confident; high doses may cause incoordination, confusion, dizziness, and nausea.

The way a drug is put into the body also shapes its effects. When you take a drug by mouth, it enters the bloodstream slowly, and its influence on the nervous system is less intense than when you bypass the gastrointestinal tract by sniffing, smoking, or injecting the drug. High doses of drugs introduced by one of these more direct routes are likely to be more harmful as well as more addicting over time.

These pharmacological facts can explain some of the variations that we see in the relationships that people form with drugs. For instance, South American Indians who chew coca leaves ordinarily swallow low doses of cocaine and do not become abusers of that stimulant. People who put much larger doses of powder cocaine in their nose or who smoke crack cocaine are much more likely to develop medical, social, and psychological problems. The abuse potential of snorting or smoking coke is far greater than the abuse potential of chewing coca. In other words, people are more likely to form a good relationship with coca than with cocaine, and this difference clearly has some basis in pharmacology.

However, the laboratory is not the real world, and pharmacology can explain only certain aspects of the complex relationships that human beings have with drugs. When people take drugs in the real world, their experiences are often not what pharmacologists would predict. The reason is that outside the laboratory other factors can completely change the effects of drugs. One such factor is known as *set;* set is what a person expects to happen when he or she takes a drug. Expectation is shaped by all of past experience — what a person has heard about the drug, read about it, seen of it, thought about it, and wants it to do. Sometimes it is not easy to find out what people expect of a drug because they may not consciously know their real feelings. A boy smoking marijuana for the first time may think that he is eager to have a new experience, whereas unconsciously he may be terrified of losing his mind or getting so stoned that he will never come down. Such unconscious fears can determine reactions to marijuana more than the actual effect of the drug.

Set can also be as important as pharmacology in shaping long-term relationships with drugs. For example, some people expect marijuana to make them relaxed and tired and so will use it only occasionally at bedtime as a sleep aid, whereas others, who feel that pot reduces their anxiety and makes it easier to relate to people, use it so frequently throughout the day that they become dependent on it.

Setting is another factor that modifies pharmacology. Setting is the environment in which a drug is used — not just the physical environment but also the social and cultural environment. During the Vietnam War many American soldiers got into the habit of smoking large amounts of the high-grade heroin that was cheap and easily available to them in Southeast Asia. They rolled it into cigarettes with tobacco or marijuana and used it primarily to escape boredom, because for many American soldiers Vietnam was, more than anything else, boring, and because heroin seems to make time pass more quickly. Pharmacologists predicted that most of these soldiers would become heroin addicts, but in fact most stopped using opiates as soon as they came home. It was the special setting of army life in Vietnam that shaped this pattern of drug use, and when people left that setting, most of them stopped easily.

Set and setting together can modify pharmacology drastically. Therefore, talking about the effects of drugs in the real world is not so simple. Effects of drugs are relative to particular people, places, and times. In ancient India marijuana was eaten for religious purposes; people used it for its effects on consciousness in socially accepted ways. In England and America during the nineteenth century, doctors gave tincture of marijuana to sick people as a remedy, and most patients never reported getting high on it, probably because they did not expect to and so ignored the psychoactive effects. In the United States in the 1920s, members of certain subcultures began smoking marijuana to feel high — a practice regarded as deviant by the dominant culture. Many early marijuana smokers panicked, and some even committed acts of violence under its influence. Today, the smoking of marijuana is accepted in many circles, and users think that it decreases aggression and hostility.

The fact that the effects of psychoactive drugs can change so much from person to person, from culture to culture, and from age to age points up the folly of calling any drug "good" or "bad." Although there is no such thing as a drug of abuse, drug abuse is real, and learning to recognize it is important. Only in analyzing people's relationships with drugs can *good* and *bad* have meaning. Some people may be upset by the notion that you can have a good relationship with a drug, but chances are that they fail to acknowledge that many socially accepted substances are, in fact, drugs.

Good relationships with drugs have four common characteristics:

1. *Recognition that the substance you are using is a drug and awareness of what it does to your body.* People who wind up in the worst relationships with drugs often have little understanding of the substances that they use. They think that coffee is just a beverage, marijuana an herb, and diet pills just "appetite suppressants." *All drugs have the potential to cause trouble unless people take care not to let their use of drugs get out of control.* A

necessary first step is to acknowledge the nature of the substances in use and to understand their effects.

2. *Experience of a useful effect of the drug over time.* People who begin to use drugs regularly often find that their early experiences with them are the best; as they use the drugs more and
   more frequently, the effects that they like seem to diminish.
   People in the worst relationships with drugs often use them
   very heavily but get the least out of them. This curious pattern
   happens with all drugs and can be very frustrating. Frequency
   of use is the critical factor in determining whether the effect
   of a drug will last over time. If the experience that you like
   from a drug begins to fade, that is a sign that you are using too
   much too often. If you ignore the warning and continue consuming the drug at the same frequency, you will begin to slide
   into a worse and worse relationship with it.

3. *Ease of separation from use of the drug.* One of the more striking
   features of a bad relationship with a drug is dependence: it
   controls you more than you control it. People in good relationships with drugs can take them or leave them. (Dependence
   on drugs is discussed at length in Chapter 12.)

4. *Freedom from adverse effects on health or behavior.* People vary in
   their susceptibility to the adverse effects of drugs. Some individuals can smoke cigarettes all their lives and never develop
   lung disease. Some people can use heroin frequently and remain physically and psychologically healthy and socially productive. Others cannot. Using drugs in ways that produce adverse effects on health and behavior, and continuing their use
   despite these effects, is the defining characteristic of drug
   abuse.

Whether a drug is legal or illegal, approved or disapproved, obtained from a physician or bought on the black market, if the user
is aware of its nature, can maintain a useful effect from it over
time, can easily separate from it, and can remain free from adverse effects, that is a good relationship with the drug.

Bad relationships with drugs begin with ignorance of the nature of the substance and loss of the desired effect with increasing frequency of use, and progress to difficulty in leaving the drug alone, with eventual impairment of health or social functioning.

Any drug can be used successfully, no matter how bad its reputation, and any drug can be abused, no matter how accepted it is. There are no good or bad drugs; there are only good and bad relationships with drugs.

SUGGESTED READING

In *Psychology of Alcohol and Other Drugs: A Research Perspective* (Thousand Oaks, Calif.: Sage, 2001), author John Jung offers a psychological perspective, synthesizing a considerable amount of research on the use of recreational drugs.

In *The Marriage of the Sun and Moon: Dispatches from the Frontiers of Consciousness* (revised edition; Boston: Houghton Mifflin, 2004), Andrew Weil presents a number of case examples of substances and techniques that can make people high. Some involve drugs such as magic mushrooms, coca leaves, and marijuana; others do not — uncontrolled laughter, Indian sweat baths, eating mangoes and hot chilies, and watching an eclipse of the sun, for example. The ways that people think about these substances and activities determine the relationships formed with them.

5. Types of Drugs

PSYCHOACTIVE DRUGS can be classified according to whether they are natural or manmade, produced by our own bodies or by plants, crude mixtures of substances or single, purified chemicals. These differences may influence the relationships that people form with drugs, and users should be aware of them.

Endogenous (In-the-Body) Drugs

The human body, especially in the brain and certain glands, makes powerful chemicals that affect our moods, thoughts, and actions. We call these substances *endogenous drugs,* using a term with Greek roots meaning "made within." Interestingly, they resemble many of the chemicals that people take to change their consciousness.

The discovery of endogenous drugs is a recent scientific breakthrough. By 1950 brain researchers had come to understand that psychoactive drugs work by fitting into special receptor sites on nerve cells, just as keys fit into locks. Only when a drug molecule combines with a receptor that fits it does it produce an effect, such as causing a nerve cell to fire an electrical impulse or preventing it from firing one. This principle is the cornerstone of current theory about drugs and the nervous system.

For example, pharmacologists learned that morphine and heroin attach to special opiate receptors on nerve cells in certain parts of the brain. But why should our brains have receptors designed to fit molecules made by poppy plants? Some researchers suggested that opiate receptors really exist for other substances made by the brain itself — molecules whose shapes happen to be similar to those of opiates. In 1975, this suggestion was confirmed with the discovery of a group of chemicals called endorphins. Endorphins are the brain's own narcotics, producing most of the effects of poppy drugs, including euphoria and reduction of pain.

Endorphins are now under intense investigation because they are likely to reveal much about the workings of our minds and bodies. People who have high tolerance for pain may produce more of these endogenous narcotics. When you wake up one day feeling high and unfazed by the problems that ordinarily get you down, your endorphin system might be in high gear. Some people may be born with an inability to make enough endorphins; they may be the people who find opiates especially pleasant and come to depend on them to cope with the pain and stress of day-to-day existence.

The discovery of endorphins also raised interesting questions. Why have the human brain and the poppy evolved chemicals with similar effects when they are so unlike each other? Is this fact a mere coincidence or does it suggest a deep relationship between people and plants that underlies the age-old inclination to experiment with vegetable drugs? And what does it say about the "naturalness" of taking drugs? It is possible that endorphins and other endogenous agents are the basis of all the highs that people experience, whether obtained with drugs or without. People who get high by meditating or running, for example, may have found ways to stimulate the production or release of their own neurochemicals.

Not only does the body make its own narcotics, it also makes representatives of most of the other categories of drugs discussed in this book. It certainly makes its own uppers in the form of adrenaline and noradrenaline. It makes its own downers in the form of serotonin and GABA (gamma-amino-butyric acid), chemicals that slow down transmission in the central nervous system. Sex hormones can be powerful antidepressants, working better than anything so far concocted in a laboratory. The body probably also makes its own psychedelics — most likely DMT (dimethyltryptamine) — since the pineal gland, deep in the brain, secretes hormones with a very similar molecular structure. And the brain has its own marijuana analog as well, a compound called anandamide.

Because the drugs that our bodies make are designed to fit exactly into receptors on nerves, they are very powerful and efficient at producing their effects. Scientists are just beginning to learn about them and will certainly have much to say on the subject in years to come. It will be interesting to know how the use of external drugs affects the production of internal ones. Perhaps regular use of a manufactured drug decreases or shuts off the production of the corresponding endogenous substance and so creates a chemical basis for dependence and addiction.

Natural Drugs

Crude Forms

Most psychoactive drugs come from plants, and there are hundreds of plants with psychoactive properties. People have put most of them to use in one part of the world or another at one time or another. Often, drug plants taste bad, are weak, or have unwanted side effects. Traditional peoples who use these plants, such as Native Americans, have come up with clever ways of preparing and ingesting them to maximize the desired effects or make them easier to take. Traditional peoples do not tamper with the chemical composition of the plants, however. For example, South American Indians have found that drying coca leaves and mixing them with ashes or other alkalis increases the stimulant effect of the leaves. To take psychedelic trips the Indians have also learned to make a powerful snuff from the resin of the Virola tree (a DMT-containing plant). In a similar way, Old World natives learned to roast coffee beans and extract them with hot water to prepare a flavorful and stimulating beverage.

Crude plant drugs contain complex mixtures of chemicals, all of which contribute to the effect of the whole. Often, the concentration of one chemical will be greater than that of any other, and that one chemical may account for the most dramatic effects of the plant. Cocaine is the main drug in coca leaves and is responsible for the numbness in the mouth and much of the stimulation that coca chewers like. In the same way, caffeine is the predominant constituent of coffee. Doctors and pharmacologists refer to these predominating chemicals as the "active principles" of the plants, which would be fine, except that the term implies that all the other constituents are inactive and unimportant.

Scientists first began to identify the active principles of well-known drug plants in the mid-1800s. They soon succeeded in isolating many and making them available in pure form. Doctors quickly began to treat patients with these purified derivatives. Today, most doctors regard green medicinal plants as old-fashioned and unscientific; they rely instead on refined white powders derived from plants. Because pharmacologists have also lost interest in plants and study only isolated active principles, they know little about how whole plants differ from refined drugs in their effects.

The relationships that people form with plants are different from those that they form with white powders. Crude natural drugs tend to be less toxic, and users tend to stay in better relationships with them over time. One reason for this difference is that plants are dilute preparations, since the active principles are combined not only with other drugs but also with inert vegetable matter. Drug plants commonly contain less than 5 percent of an active principle. (Coca rarely has more than 0.5 percent cocaine.) By contrast, refined preparations may approach 100 percent purity.

In addition, crude plants usually go into the body through the mouth and stomach, whereas purified chemicals can be put into the bloodstream more directly, such as by snorting, smoking, or injecting. (You can't snort a coca leaf.) Harmful effects, both immediate and long-term, are more likely to appear when people put drugs directly into their bloodstream without giving their body a chance to process them.

Finally, the many other compounds in drug plants — often a single plant will contain twenty or more active components — may modify the active principles, making them safer or softening their harsher actions on the body. These safety factors and modifiers are lost when the active principles are isolated from the crude drugs that nature provides.

Natural drugs in whole plant form are the safest types of drugs. They always have lower potential for abuse. If people choose to take drugs, they would be wise to use natural plant forms in order to give themselves the best chance of avoiding problems.

Refined Forms

Morphine, cocaine, and mescaline are all examples of drugs that occur in plants but are commonly available in refined form as white powders, sold both legally and illegally. Some of them, such as mescaline, can easily be synthesized in laboratories, but even when they are, we can still call them natural drugs because the molecules already exist in nature. Others, such as cocaine and morphine, have more complex molecular structures. Chemists can make them in laboratories, but it is not cost efficient to do so. All the cocaine and morphine on the black market and in pharmacies is extracted from coca leaves and opium poppies.

Extraction and purification of some plant drugs is long and complicated, requiring sophisticated techniques and equipment. In other cases, the process is so simple that unskilled people can do it in the kitchen. Black-market cocaine is usually made in primitive jungle factories; of course, it is likely to contain many impurities.

Whether natural drugs are manufactured by chemists or extracted from plants, they may be safer than drugs that nature never thought of, because natural drugs interact more smoothly with the body's own chemistry. Since their structures tend to be closer to those of endogenous drugs, the effects of natural drugs and endogenous drugs tend to be similar. As we have noted, however, it is important to distinguish natural drugs in the dilute form of crude plants from refined powders with much higher toxicity and abuse potential.

Semisynthetic Drugs

Pharmacologists often take refined natural drugs and change their chemical structure to vary their properties. A very simple change is to combine an insoluble drug from a plant with an acid to make a water-soluble salt. In this way the "freebase" form of co-caine, which is usually smoked because it will not dissolve, is turned into cocaine hydrochloride, a water-soluble compound that can be inhaled or injected.

A slightly more complicated transformation is the addition of chemical groups to a natural drug molecule to make it stronger. At the end of the nineteenth century, German chemists created as-pirin by adding an acetic acid group to a natural pain-relieving chemical found in the bark of some willow trees. Native Ameri-cans drank willow-bark tea to treat headaches and rheumatism, but aspirin is a more powerful pain reliever than willow bark. (It is also much more toxic.) A similar addition of two acetic acid groups to morphine turns it into heroin, a similar but more potent drug. That is, it takes less heroin than morphine to produce the same effect.

These transformations of natural drugs result in new sub-stances called semisynthetic drugs. Chemists like to make semi-synthetic drugs because it is easier to play with an existing mole-cule than to start from scratch. Sometimes their experiments only intensify the action of the original compound, as in the examples of aspirin and heroin, while in other cases, the results are com-pletely novel. LSD (lysergic acid diethylamide) is an example of a semisynthetic drug with novel properties. It was made from a nat-ural chemical in a fungus called ergot that attacks grasses and grains, but the original chemical (lysergic acid) is toxic and has lit-tle psychoactivity.

The ability of chemists to create new drugs from natural compounds raises an old argument about whether human beings should tamper with nature. We think that people are meant to interact with the natural world and modify its creations. In fact, people can improve on nature. A fine example is the development of excellent varieties of fruits and vegetables from unimpressive wild species. The issue for us is whether the results of the manipulations are beneficial or harmful. Plant selection and breeding to enhance flavor and nutrition are clearly worthwhile. On the other hand, the production of square, hard, tasteless tomatoes to facilitate mass packing and shipping is inspired by greed rather than a desire to benefit humanity.

In the same way, when chemists tinker with natural drugs, they should attempt to maximize desirable qualities. Extreme potency is not necessarily desirable, because it often goes hand in hand with great toxicity. We pay a high price today for our rejection of natural medicines in favor of potent chemicals. The tendency of pharmacologists and doctors to regard more potent drugs as better drugs encourages the use of dangerous derivatives of plants, when often the milder, natural originals would do as well.

Synthetic Drugs

Wholly synthetic drugs are made from scratch in the laboratory and do not occur naturally. Valium, PCP (phencyclidine), and secobarbital (Seconal) are examples. It may be that synthetic drugs are the most dangerous of all and the hardest to form a good relationship with, but it is risky to make such sweeping judgments. Very recently, researchers discovered Valium receptors in the human brain, leading them to believe that the body must produce some internal analog to that completely synthetic tranquilizer. Did the chemists who created Valium in a laboratory hit upon that molecule only by chance? Has Valium become so popular because its effect resembles that of an endogenous substance? Or might Valium receptors have developed in the brain in response to use of the drug? It is interesting to speculate on these questions, even though science may never be able to answer them.

In the following pages we describe all the psychoactive drugs that people are likely to encounter, both those that are legal and those that are not. We discuss them category by category, explaining how they work and what their benefits and dangers are. In any category, such as stimulants, some drugs may be natural — in crude or refined form — some may be semisynthetic, and some totally synthetic. We do not dwell on these differences but encourage the reader to keep in mind that dilute, natural forms of substances are always safer and may give users the best chance to build stable relationships with the drugs that they take.

SUGGESTED READING

There is no good book on the different types of drugs discussed in this chapter or on the new discoveries about endogenous drugs.

Guide to Psychoactive Drugs by Richard Seymour and David E. Smith (New York: Harrington Park Press, 1987) is a good, readable reference book. See also *Uppers, Downers, All Arounders: Physical and Mental Effects of Psychoactive Drugs* by Darryl S. Inaba and William E. Cohen (Ashland, Oreg.: Cris Productions, 1997).

Buzzed: The Straight Facts About the Most Used and Abused Drugs from Alcohol to Ecstasy by Scott Swartzwelder et al. (New York: W. W. Norton, 1998) is a succinct and clear guide to the often overcomplicated subject of neurochemistry. The book is divided into twelve sections covering all types of drugs.

6. Stimulants

STIMULANTS ARE DRUGS that make people feel more alert and energetic by activating or exciting the nervous system. There are many stimulant drugs in current use; some are plants found in nature, others are chemicals made in the laboratory. These different drugs produce somewhat different effects, lasting for varying lengths of time, but all of them raise the energy level of the nervous system in roughly the same way.

The individual nerves in our bodies communicate with each other both electrically and chemically. A nerve impulse is an electric discharge that moves quickly along the fiber of a nerve cell. The fiber may end at a muscle, a gland, or another nerve cell, but there is always a tiny space between the end of the nerve fiber and the next cell. To bridge this gap, the nerve fiber releases small amounts of powerful chemicals called neurotransmitters that affect the next cell. Some neurotransmitters are strong stimulants that cause muscle cells to contract, gland cells to secrete, and other nerve cells to fire off electrical discharges. The most common stimulant neurotransmitter is a chemical called noradrenaline, or norepinephrine. This chemical is closely related to the hormone adrenaline (or epinephrine), which is produced by our adrenal glands. (*Adrenal* is a Latin word meaning "on the kidney," because

> Thank God for tea! What would the world do without tea?
> — how did it exist? I am glad I was not born before tea.
>
> **— Sydney Smith (1771–1845), English clergyman, writer, and wit**

the adrenal glands sit on top of the kidneys like little caps. *Epinephros* means the same thing in Greek. In America the Parke-Davis pharmaceutical company succeeded in registering Adrenalin as a trademark for its brand of adrenal hormone, which is why American scientists generally use the more cumbersome words *epinephrine* and *norepinephzine*. We prefer the Latin form.)

Stimulant drugs work by causing nerve fibers to release noradrenaline and other stimulating neurotransmitters. Although different stimulants bring about this release in different ways, the end result is always the same: the release of more stimulating neurotransmitters. So the stimulation that people feel when they take stimulant drugs is simply a result of the chemical energy of the body's going to work in the nervous system. The drug just makes the body expend this energy sooner and in greater quantity than it would ordinarily.

This release of chemical energy in the form of noradrenaline causes certain predictable changes in the mind and body. It makes a person feel wakeful, alert, and, often, happy. It makes the heart beat faster and may cause the blood pressure to rise. Because it produces changes in blood flow, the fingertips and tip of the nose may become cold. It gives a feeling of butterflies in the stomach and may cause a laxative effect.

Some of these changes are mediated by a branch of the nervous system called the sympathetic nervous system. The main function of the sympathetic nervous system is to respond to emergencies by preparing the body for fight or flight. It does so by shutting down nonessential functions and speeding up vital ones. The sympathetic nervous system relies on noradrenaline as its chemical messenger.

Noradrenaline acts in many of the same ways as adrenaline, the hormone secreted by the adrenal glands, also in response to emergencies. Experiences that cause the adrenals to secrete adrenaline into the bloodstream produce feelings very much like those of stimulant drugs. The rush of excitement during a roller coaster ride, for example, may feel a lot like the effect of a dose of amphetamine, and no doubt both these techniques are popular for the same reason — because they give people a sense of increased mental and physical energy and make them feel, temporarily at least, more alive.

In recent years, scientists have begun to find out many interesting things about biorhythms, the cycles by which our vital processes wax and wane. The most obvious daily biorhythm is that of sleeping and waking. Production of hormones and neurotransmitters has its own ups and downs, and these cycles probably explain why people feel naturally stimulated at certain times and naturally lethargic at others. A common pattern is to feel energetic and able to concentrate well in the morning but to become tired and mentally sluggish in the late afternoon.

One reason that stimulant drugs are popular is that they give us temporary control over the rhythms of wakefulness and the ups and downs of mood. If you have a mental task to do at 3 P.M., when your brain wants to rest, you can mobilize it to concentrate by taking a stimulant drug and thereby forcing your nervous system to release some of its stored-up chemical energy. Or if you have to drive a long distance at night when your whole nervous system is ready for sleep, you can stay awake by putting a stimulant into your body. Or if you are feeling depressed when you have to go out and meet important people, a stimulant might brighten your mood for a while.

Another reason that people like stimulants is that they suppress hunger, making it possible to think about something other than food and concentrate better on the task at hand. Not eating, moreover, tends to further increase one's energy and sense of alertness. The reason that stimulant drugs suppress hunger probably has to do with the preparation of the body for emergencies. In emergencies, all digestive functions become nonessential compared to such processes as blood circulation and speed of muscular response. Under stress, therefore, the body shifts energy away from the stomach and intestines to the brain, heart, and blood vessels.

Because the nerves and muscles receive more attention under

the effect of stimulants, these drugs may improve certain kinds of physical and mental performance for a time. They may enable people to concentrate longer and better or to perform physical work more efficiently and with greater endurance. This probably explains why these drugs are especially popular with students and athletes.

Of course, stimulants do not affect everyone in the same way; some people find the effects of these drugs unpleasant, just as some people find roller coaster rides unpleasant. Far from making everyone cheerful and alert, these drugs make many people anxious, jittery, and unable to sit still. Some people are so sensitive to stimulants that they cannot sleep at all, even twelve hours after taking a small dose. Others get such distressing symptoms as heart palpitations, diarrhea, and urinary frequency and urgency. Instead of automatically improving physical and mental performance, stimulants sometimes just make people do poor work faster. There are famous (probably apocryphal) stories of college students who, under the influence of amphetamines, wrote what they imagined to be brilliant final exams, only to find later that they had written the same line over and over or scribbled the whole exam on one illegible page.

Still, at first glance, stimulants sound attractive: they can make you feel alert, happy, wakeful, energetic, strong, and resistant to hunger, boredom, and fatigue. But one of life's basic rules is that you never get something for nothing (or, there's no such thing as a free lunch), and stimulants are no exception to this rule.

The most serious problems with stimulant drugs result from the way they work. For, instead of miraculously delivering free gifts of cosmic energy, stimulants merely force the body to give up some of its own energy reserves. So, when the effect of a stimulant wears off, the body is left with less energy than usual and must replenish its supplies.

People experience this depletion of energy as a "down" or "low" state, marked by the very same feelings that they take stimulants to avoid, namely, sleepiness, lethargy, laziness, mental fatigue, and depression. The price that you pay for the good feeling that a stimulant gives you is a not-so-good feeling when the stimulant wears off.

If you are willing to pay this price and let your body recharge itself, there is nothing wrong with using stimulants now and then. The trouble is that many people are not willing to let their bodies readjust; they want to feel good again right away, so they take another dose of the drug. It's very easy to fall into a pattern of using stimulants all the time in order to avoid the down feeling that follows the initial up.

Unfortunately, when stimulants are used in this way, they quickly produce dependence. People who regularly take stimulants find that they cannot function normally without them. They need them just to open their eyes in the morning, move their bowels, work, or do any of the tasks of everyday life. Without stimulants these people just don't feel like doing much of anything.

Kinds of Stimulants

Coffee and Other Caffeine-Containing Plants

Caffeine, the most popular natural stimulant, is found in a number of plants throughout the world. The drug was first isolated from coffee in 1821 and was named for that plant, but the effects of coffee and caffeine differ. In many ways, coffee seems to be more powerful than refined caffeine or other caffeine-containing plants.

A shrubby tree native to Ethiopia, coffee is now cultivated in many tropical countries throughout the world. Each of its bright red fruits, called cherries, contains two seeds, or beans. The raw beans are gray-green and odorless, but when roasted they turn dark brown and develop their characteristic aroma and flavor. Legend has it that coffee was first discovered long ago by Ethiopian nomads who noticed that their domestic animals became frisky

> In the morning, I drink two cups of coffee. If I don't, I feel
> irritable. If I drink three cups, I get a little speedy, but with
> two I feel just about right.
>
> — thirty-nine-year-old man, college administrator

after eating the fruit of the trees. When people tried eating the
seeds, they got frisky too, and eventually they learned to make a
flavorful drink from the roasted seeds.

More than a thousand years ago, groups of Muslims in the
Middle East began using coffee in religious rituals and ceremonies. Groups of men would meet one night a week, drink large
amounts of coffee, and stay up all night praying and chanting.
These mystics confined their use of coffee to occasional ceremonies, but as coffee became more widely known, other people began to use it, not for religious reasons but just because they liked
its stimulant effect. When people started to drink coffee every
day in large amounts, many of them found that they couldn't stop.

When coffee first came to Europe in the seventeenth century, it
stirred up great opposition as a new and unapproved drug. Authorities tried to prohibit its use, but of course their efforts were to
no avail; coffee soon established itself there and all over the world.
Coffee houses sprang up in all European cities, and whole populations became dependent on the drug almost overnight. Johann
Sebastian Bach is rumored to have been a coffee addict. He ex-
tolled the virtues of the new drink in his famous Coffee Cantata.
The French writer Honoré de Balzac could not work without coffee. He drank larger and larger amounts of a brew that was so
strong that it looked like thick soup; then he complained of the
stomach cramps that coffee gave him.

Today, coffee is a thoroughly approved drug — so approved, in
fact, that many people who drink it regularly are surprised to learn

> Far beyond all other pleasures, rarer than jewels or trea-
> sures, sweeter than grape from the vine. Yes! Yes! Greatest
> of pleasures! Coffee, coffee, how I love its flavor, and if
> you would win my favor, yes! Yes! let me have coffee, let
> me have my coffee strong.
>
> — from the Coffee Cantata, by Johann Sebastian Bach (1685–1750)

that it is a drug at all, let alone a powerful drug that can cause dependence and illness.

The truth is that coffee is a strong stimulant, one that is hard on
certain parts of the body. It is irritating to the stomach, for example, and many people who drink a lot of it have indigestion most of
the time. (In the United States, where people regularly consume
coffee in large quantities, there are nearly as many brands of antacids as there are brands of coffee.) It is irritating to the bladder,
too, especially in women, and is a frequent cause of urinary complaints. Coffee also makes many people shaky by upsetting the
delicate balance between nerves and muscles. It is a common
cause of headaches, heart palpitations, anxiety, and insomnia.

Today, dependence on coffee is very common in Western society. Many regular users cannot think clearly in the morning until
they have had their first cup. Without it, they can't concentrate,
move their bowels, or do their work. Also, they suffer real withdrawal symptoms if they stop using coffee suddenly. The withdrawal reaction begins twenty-four to thirty-six hours after the last
dose. Symptoms are lethargy, irritability, and a distinctive throbbing (vascular) headache that is often severe. Nausea and vomiting may occur. These symptoms will last from thirty-six to sev-
enty-two hours. They disappear rapidly if the user takes caffeine in
any form. Such problems all come from using coffee so frequently
that the body never gets a chance to replenish its stores of chemical energy and comes to rely more and more on the external drug.

Coffee and caffeine have been suspected of causing birth defects. So far, the evidence is not conclusive, but pregnant women should remember that coffee and caffeine are drugs and that they should not consume them in large amounts. Coffee and caffeine may also raise serum cholesterol, increasing the risk of heart attack. The evidence for this effect remains contradictory. On the other hand, coffee may offer protection from pancreatic cancer, a rare and deadly disease.

Note that decaffeinated coffee is not inert. In addition to small amounts of caffeine (enough to stimulate sensitive individuals), it contains other active substances from the coffee bean that can be irritating to the nervous, gastrointestinal, cardiovascular, and urinary systems. This is true of water-processed decaf as well as the less safe solvent-extracted brands, which may contain residues of toxic chemicals.

Other caffeine beverages don't seem to be as powerful or as toxic as coffee — even though they may contain as much caffeine or equivalent drugs. Tea is not nearly so irritating to the body as coffee, and cases of dependence on tea are less common in our society. Of course, tea is a stimulant, and if you drink it in large amounts or make it strong enough, you can get powerful effects, including jitteriness and insomnia. In England, tea drinking has been a national pastime and habit since the early seventeenth century, when it was introduced from Asia. Tea addiction is not uncommon in England, Ireland, and Asia. Japanese people drink green tea throughout the day. In addition, they conduct tea ceremonies, elaborate rituals built around the consumption of *matcha,*

We had a kettle; we let it leak.
Our not repairing it made it worse.
We haven't had any tea for a week . . .
The bottom is out of the Universe.

— "Natural Theology," by Rudyard Kipling (1865–1936)

a special powdered green tea that is whipped with water into a bitter, frothy beverage. This strong form of tea was developed in Zen Buddhist monasteries to help monks stay awake during long hours of meditation.

A great deal of recent medical research has documented the health benefits of tea, especially green tea, which is a rich source of antioxidants that may lower cholesterol and help prevent cancer and other chronic diseases. The main antioxidant in tea is EGCG (epigallocatechin gallate). It is highest in the least processed forms of tea, such as Chinese white tea and Japanese green, lower in leaves that have been oxidized to change their color and flavor, like oolong and black tea. Another interesting compound in tea is L-theanine, which causes "alert relaxation." (It is now available as a dietary supplement.) This compound may modify the effect of caffeine, which is why most people find even strong tea to be less "jangling" than coffee.

Cola is a caffeine-containing seed, or nut, from a tropical tree, the cola tree. In some African countries, cola nuts are so valuable that they are used as money. The nuts have a bitter, aromatic taste, and people chew them for their stimulating effect. Bottled cola drinks have very little cola nut in them and do not taste like cola nuts at all. Though they do contain caffeine, it is usually synthetic caffeine or caffeine extracted from coffee or tea. These soft drinks are also drugs, and people can become dependent on them, as with coffee. Also, they contain a lot of sugar.

The combination of sugar and caffeine seems to be especially habit-forming. Many people drink enormous amounts of cola, and although they may think that they are merely quenching their thirst, they are also consuming calories and enough sugar to damage their teeth (and upset their metabolism), not to mention large doses of caffeine. (Diet colas eliminate the sugar but not the caffeine.) Like other stimulants, cola drinks are not unhealthy if used in moderation; people who like them should just be aware of their nature and their potential for abuse. Parents especially should remember that so-called soft drinks are actually drugs that can affect the health and mood of their children. (The popularity of stimulating cola drinks has led manufacturers to add caffeine to some other flavors of carbonated beverages. Drinks so fortified must list caffeine as an ingredient. If you do not want to take drugs with your soda, you should make a habit of reading the information on bottles and cans.)

In other parts of the world, people use a number of less well-known caffeine plants. The national drink of Brazil is *guaraná* (pronounced gwah-rah-NAH), made from the seeds of a jungle shrub. It contains more caffeine than coffee and is often made into sweet carbonated drinks. Tablets of *guaraná* powder have appeared in health food stores in the United States under such brand names as ZOOM and ZING, and more recently many brands of *guaraná*-based energy drinks have joined the tablets; the drinks are marketed as new organic stimulants from the Amazon rain forest.

In Argentina, the most popular caffeine drink is maté (pronounced mah-TAY), which is made from the leaves of a holly plant. Some kinds of maté taste like smoky tea. Maté leaves can be bought in health food stores and tea shops and are ingredients in some herbal tea mixtures, such as Celestial Seasonings' Morning Thunder. Packages of maté sometimes misrepresent the product as a caffeine-free herbal tea.

One of the most famous sources of caffeine is chocolate, also made from the seeds of a tropical tree. (The tree is called cacao [pronounced cah-COW], and its seeds are cacao beans, or cocoa beans. The fat in them is cocoa butter. White chocolate is just cocoa butter mixed with sugar. The roasted ground-up beans, with most of the fat removed, are cocoa. Regular chocolate is made by adding extra fat to roasted ground-up beans.) Chocolate, which contains a lot of fat and is very bitter, must be mixed with sugar to make it palatable. Chocolate, too, contains a stimulating drug, and cases of chocolate dependence are easy to find. You probably know a few "chocoholics." People who regularly consume chocolate or go on chocolate-eating binges may not realize that they are in-

> Five years ago, hoping to kick a chocolate habit that was
> significantly affecting my life, I enrolled in a program at
> the Shick Center for the Control of Smoking, Alcoholism,
> and Overeating, in Los Angeles. I was then thirty-three.
> I could not remember the last time I had managed to
> get through a whole day without eating chocolate in
> one form or another, usually in quantities most people
> would regard as excessive, if not appalling . . . Frankly,
> I am mystified by what happened and to this day cannot
> explain it. Being addicted to chocolate was so much a
> part of my definition of myself that it constantly amazes
> me to think that I am now free of it.
>
> — thirty-eight-year-old woman, social worker

volved with a drug, but their consumption usually follows the
same sort of pattern as with coffee, tea, and cola drinks.

Chocolate contains only a small amount of caffeine but has a lot
of theobromine, a close relative with similar effects. By itself,
theobromine cannot account for all aspects of chocolate addiction,
because chocolate addiction looks different from other forms of
stimulant dependence. Most chocoholics are women, and many of
them crave chocolate most intensely just before their menstrual
periods. Women who develop an addictive relationship with chocolate usually eat it in cyclic binges rather than continually and often say that it acts on them like an instant antidepressant. As there
is no reason to think that theobromine affects men and women
differently, other components of chocolate must be involved. Very
little research has been done on chocolate, so no one knows for
sure.

Cacao was known to the ancient Aztecs, who considered it a sacred plant and used it in religious rituals. Dark chocolate is a rich

source of health-protective antioxidants, like green tea and red wine. It has heart-protective effects and may actually help lower cholesterol. In moderation, chocolate is a pleasant and interesting addition to the diet, but overuse may not be wise, especially since the combination of sugar, fat, and drugs can be so habit-forming. People who tend to gain weight easily should be especially careful about their intake of chocolate.

Coca and Cocaine

Coca, a shrub native to the hot, humid valleys of the eastern slopes of the Andes, has been cultivated by the Indians of South America for thousands of years. Today, the plant is legal in Peru and Bolivia, where millions of Indians still chew coca leaves every day as a stimulant and medicine. (Coca, by the way, is not related to cocoa.)

Coca contains fourteen drugs, the most important of which is cocaine. The other drugs are present in smaller amounts and seem to modify the stimulating effect of the cocaine. In addition, coca leaves contain many vitamins and minerals that are probably important in the diets of Indians who use the leaves. There are several varieties of coca: some taste like green tea, some like wintergreen. Coca users put dried leaves in their mouth and work them into a large wad. They suck on this wad for thirty minutes or so, swallowing the juices and then spitting out the residue. To get an effect from coca, the user must add a tiny amount of some alkali, such as lime (the powdered mineral) or ashes, to the wad of leaves.

After a few minutes of chewing coca, the user's mouth and tongue become numb; then people begin to experience the usual effects of a stimulant. Unlike coffee, coca soothes the stomach and doesn't produce jitteriness. It may also be more powerful than caffeine in producing a good mood.

In the late 1800s, coca became very popular in Europe and America in the form of tonics and wines. Coca-Cola began as one

Had drugs been decriminalized seventeen years ago, crack would never have been invented. It was invented because the high cost of illegal drugs made it profitable to provide a cheaper version.

— economist Milton Friedman, writing in the *Wall Street Journal*, September 7, 1989

of these early preparations. At the same time, scientists isolated cocaine from the leaves and made it available to doctors in the form of a pure white powder. As the first local anesthetic, cocaine revolutionized surgery, especially eye operations, which had always been terribly painful and difficult. In the 1880s, doctors began to prescribe cocaine for all sorts of medical problems, including dependence on opiates and alcohol. It soon became apparent that this kind of treatment was not a good idea, because many patients suffered ill effects from cocaine, and many became dependent on it. So, in the early 1900s, laws were passed to prevent the widespread use of coca and cocaine. The Coca-Cola Company took cocaine out of its drink (it still contains a drug-free extract of the leaves as a flavor). Other coca products swiftly disappeared from the shelves of drugstores. Safer local anesthetics were invented in laboratories, and today doctors use cocaine only for certain operations in the eye, nose, throat, and mouth.

In the hundred years since Congress restricted the use of coca, a huge black market has developed to supply cocaine to the many people who like the feeling that it gives. All illegal cocaine comes from leaves grown and processed in South America. It is always cut (diluted) with various substances before reaching consumers here. Most people snort cocaine, that is, they snuff the powder up their noses. Used in this way, the stimulant effects come on very fast, are very intense, and are very short-lived. Some people shoot cocaine, that is, inject it intravenously, which gives even faster, more intense, and shorter effects (see Chapter 12 for the health problems related to intravenous drug use), and some people use water pipes to smoke a special form of cocaine called freebase. Crack cocaine is a newer, smokable form of the drug marketed as small pellets. It first appeared in the mid-1980s, and crack use quickly reached epidemic proportions in cities throughout America. Smoking puts cocaine into the bloodstream even faster than intravenous injection and gives similar effects — very intense and very brief. Few people take cocaine by mouth, even though it works and is actually much safer that way.

Coca and cocaine are very different, and the difference shows how it is easier to form good relationships with natural drugs than with isolated and refined ones.

Coca leaves contain low concentrations of cocaine (usually only 0.5 percent), in combination with other drugs that modify its effects in a good way; they also contain valuable nutrients. The cocaine is highly diluted by inactive leaf material. What's more, getting stimulation from coca takes work: you have to chew a mouthful of leaves for half an hour. In this natural form, small amounts of cocaine enter the bloodstream slowly through the mouth and stomach.

Relatively pure street cocaine may contain 60 percent of the drug, which, when it is put directly into the nose, lungs, or veins, enters the bloodstream all at once. The stimulation, or "rush," is therefore very intense, but it lasts only a short time, usually disappearing within fifteen to thirty minutes. Then the user may crash, feeling tired, sluggish, unhappy. Because cocaine can make people feel so good for so short a time and not so good immediately thereafter, users tend to go on using it, trying to get back the good feeling. Many people can't leave this drug alone if they have it, even though all they get from it after a while is the unpleasant effects characteristic of all stimulants used in excess: anxiety, insomnia, and general feelings of discomfort. Besides, snorting too much powder cocaine irritates the nose, while smoking crack may be bad for the lungs and is even more likely to lead to overuse and a stubborn habit.

Indians in South America, on the other hand, rarely have any problems with coca leaf. They can take it or leave it, continue to get good effects from it over time, and use the stimulation to help them work or socialize. They also use it as a medicine for a variety of illnesses, especially digestive ones. Among South American Indians, there is little abuse of coca leaf.

Use and abuse of cocaine have skyrocketed in recent years, provoking much public alarm. Sensational news stories about crack, with graphic descriptions of inner-city crack houses and impaired "crack babies" born to addicted mothers, led directly to escalation of the current war on drugs. For drug warriors, crack became the new devil drug, so dangerous as to justify the most repressive measures.

In their enthusiasm to fight cocaine these crusaders often exaggerated its dangers, at least its physical toxicity. Both powder and crack cocaine can increase the workload of the heart and cause irregular heartbeats, but death from cocaine is rare, and the body has a great capacity to metabolize and eliminate the drug from its system. Actually, what drug education should emphasize are the psychological and social dangers of cocaine.

First of all, the addictiveness of this stimulant is great. (Smoking crack is as addictive as smoking cigarettes.) Cocaine addiction almost always interferes with social and economic functioning, since addicts often alienate their family and friends, lose their jobs, and spend phenomenal amounts of money on their habits ($15,000 a year and more). They become paranoid, isolated, and depressed, unable to stop thinking about their next dose. Treatment of this addictive behavior is difficult, time-consuming, and costly.

Occasional snorting of powder cocaine in social situations is probably not harmful for most people, but everyone should be aware that the possibility of using this drug to excess is very real and that excessive cocaine use can wreck a person's life. It is even more difficult to limit the intake of crack cocaine to levels compatible with good physical and emotional health.

Once the drug of choice of yuppies, socialites, and dot-com millionaires, cocaine has now diffused through much of American society, although it has been replaced in some communities by methamphetamine, which is cheaper and gives longer-lasting stimulation. Nevertheless, the production of coca in Peru and Bolivia and the refining of leaves into cocaine in Colombia continue unabated, as does the American effort to eradicate the plant.

It seems a shame that the laws and policies on drugs in our society have led to the disappearance of coca, along with knowledge of its uses and benefits. At the same time, by outlawing something that many people want, legislators have made it profitable to smuggle the concentrated drug and so have encouraged the growth of a vast black market in cocaine. The American-led war against the cocaine trade has caused incalculable social, political, economic, and ecological devastation in the producing countries of South America.

Amphetamines and Related Drugs

Amphetamines are synthetic stimulants that were invented in Germany in the 1930s. Their chemical structures resemble those of adrenaline and noradrenaline, the body's own stimulants. The effects of amphetamines resemble those of cocaine but are much longer lasting. A single oral dose of amphetamine usually stimulates the body for at least four hours.

Amphetamines are more toxic than cocaine and, when abused, cause worse problems. The body has a great capacity to metabolize and eliminate cocaine: the liver can detoxify a lethal dose of cocaine every thirty minutes. It cannot handle amphetamines as efficiently. At the same time, people can establish a stable relationship with amphetamines more easily than they can with cocaine, probably because the intensely pleasurable but very short effect of cocaine is more seductive and invites repetitive dosing.

For many years after the invention of amphetamines, they were tolerated and their use was even encouraged by authorities. Soldiers in World War II received rations of amphetamines to make

I decided to try and make up for lost time by staying up all night to study for my European history exam, but by midnight the text was blurring before my eyes ... An upperclassman took pity on me and offered me a green-and-white capsule along with the promise that my drowsiness would be cured by taking it. I took it without a second thought and within half an hour or so found myself studying like mad. Not only was I completely engrossed in European history, I felt exhilarated; I was actually enjoying myself ... I got an A on my history exam — as I was sure I had — and have been involved, to some extent, with amphetamines ever since.

— forty-two-year-old woman, writer

them march longer and fight better. The governments of several countries, among them the Soviet Union, experimented with giving amphetamines to factory workers, hoping to make them more productive (which, in the long run, they failed to do). Doctors in this country have prescribed them in great quantity for even more questionable reasons.

In the 1950s and 1960s, the U.S. pharmaceutical industry manufactured enormous quantities of amphetamines (many of which turned up on the black market). The companies urged doctors to prescribe their products for depressed housewives and people with weight problems.

There are a number of different amphetamines, but all have the same basic effect. Plain amphetamine (Benzedrine) was the first to become popular. Dextroamphetamine (Dexedrine) and methamphetamine (Methedrine) are effective in lower doses but otherwise are similar to the parent compound. A few other drugs — methylphenidate (Ritalin), for example — resemble amphetamines in effect, even though they have a different chemical structure. And a new class of "wakefulness promoting agents" has just appeared; the first on the market is modafinil (Provigil). Originally developed to keep military personnel awake while on duty, it is now used to treat narcolepsy, a medical condition marked by excessive sleepiness. A few users of amphetamines tell us that they would use modafinil only if they couldn't get their preferred stimulants.

Today, we know that regular use of amphetamines, especially by people who are neurotic, depressed, or fat, is not a good idea. Not only do the drugs fail to help their problems, they often complicate matters by creating another kind of dependence. Since the 1970s most cases of amphetamine abuse have involved legally manufactured and prescribed drugs. At about the same time, criticism of the promotional practices of pharmaceutical companies and of the prescribing practices of physicians brought about severe restrictions on the medical use of these compounds. Today, amphetamines can be prescribed for only a few conditions.

One of the more controversial uses still permitted is the control of attention deficit hyperactivity disorder (ADHD) in children. For reasons that scientists do not yet understand, amphetamines (and other stimulants) have a calming effect on many children. Unfortunately, the diagnosis of ADHD often is applied to children who simply misbehave or don't pay attention in school. Giving them amphetamines not only fails to get to the root of the problem, it introduces young people to powerful drugs and encourages among adults the false notion that all of life's problems can be solved by taking pills. Stimulants can be life changing for some children with ADHD, but it cannot be good for so many young people to be on these drugs. One popular drug for ADHD is Adderall, a combination of dextroamphetamine and methamphetamine. Extra-long-acting forms of these stimulants are now popular with parents and doctors. But the intense appetite suppression that they cause can actually interfere with nutrition and growth in young children.

Given the restrictions on the legal supplies and uses of amphetamines, black markets in them grew, and, as so often happens, this change promoted abuse. In the days of legal pills, most users took them by mouth. Today, many people snort powdered amphetamines like cocaine, smoke them like crack, and even inject them intravenously.

Intravenous use of amphetamines first appeared in the late 1960s. Young "speed freaks" who fell into this pattern of use experienced very bad effects on their bodies and minds. After only a few weeks, they became emaciated and generally unhealthy; they stayed up for days on end, then "crashed" into a stupor. They became jumpy, paranoid, and even psychotic. Members of the drug subculture itself recognized the dangers of shooting amphetamines and warned people about it with the phrase "speed kills."

But the most noteworthy change in the distribution and use of amphetamines has been the explosive popularity of methamphetamine, known as "meth" or "crank." The crystalline, smokable form of it is called "ice" or "crystal." Heavy ice smokers go on binges that can last for days, a practice known as "tweaking" or "amping." Crystal meth is now the illegal drug of choice in much of rural America, its use rampant in economically depressed farm communities of the Midwest and West. A great increase in property crime has followed in the wake of this epidemic. Smoking crystal meth is as hazardous as injecting it.

It is easy to make methamphetamine from such ingredients as agricultural fertilizer, and large numbers of meth labs have appeared all over the country, especially in less populated areas, where the strong odors resulting from cooking the drug are less likely to draw attention. It is not uncommon to hear of disastrous accidents during meth production — explosions and serious injuries. Once an area has been used as a meth lab, it is an environmental hazard, very costly to clean up.

Note that many people are able to use amphetamines without problems, especially if they take them orally, moderately, and purposefully. For example, some college students use them to study for or take exams. Some writers take them to work. Truckers and other drivers sometimes take them for long-distance travel on highways, especially at night. Athletes, such as football players, sometimes use them to play big games. Actors and dancers take them occasionally to perform. Used in this way, amphetamines do not usually cause physical harm, especially if people rest afterward. Problems arise when people take amphetamines all the time, just because they like the feeling of stimulation, especially if they snort, smoke, or shoot amphetamines.

"Look-alike" Drugs

As the regulation of medical prescription of amphetamines tightened up, a flood of bogus products appeared. Called look-alikes, they are tablets and capsules that are made to look like pharmaceutical amphetamines but that contain no controlled substances. Some are legally manufactured for over-the-counter sale in drug and health food stores; others appear in head shops or are sold by mail order or on the Internet or street.

Look-alikes contain caffeine, ephedrine, phenylpropanolamine, or synephrine, either singly or in combination. Ephedrine is a natural stimulant with a chemical structure that resembles adrenaline, but ephedrine produces more anxiety and less euphoria than amphetamines. It occurs in a desert shrub and has been used as a treatment for asthma (see page 63). Phenylpropanolamine (PPA) is a synthetic drug that once was added to many cold remedies as a nasal decongestant. Not long ago it was also an ingredient in a number of over-the-counter diet pills. Now that PPA and ephedrine are banned, manufacturers have turned to synephrine, which is obtained from bitter orange. Look for a ban on it in the near future.

Look-alike drugs have received much bad publicity. They are accused of killing some people by causing strokes and disturbances of their heartbeat. There is no hard evidence to support this, but people with high blood pressure or a history of heart irregularities should be wary of them (as they should be of all stimulants).

> Several years ago, I fell madly in love with an ex-smoker, a man who, though broad-minded in other respects, was a fanatic on the subject of cigarettes . . . I had always thought I'd be able to kick my addiction to cigarettes for someone I loved. That assumption turned out to be wrong. In the end, when forced to choose between love and cigarettes, I chose cigarettes. It was that simple. I did make one resolution at the time, which I have stuck to ever since. It was that I would never again become involved with a man who does not smoke cigarettes.
>
> **— forty-one-year-old woman, teacher**

Tobacco and Nicotine

Tobacco is one of the most powerful stimulant plants known, and nicotine — its active principle — is one of the most toxic of all drugs. An average cigar contains enough nicotine to kill several people.

When tobacco is smoked, burning it destroys most of the nicotine. (To kill people with a cigar, you'd have to soak the cigar in water till it turned dark, then make people drink the liquid.) Nicotine is so strong and dangerous that the body quickly develops tolerance for it to protect itself. If someone begins smoking regularly, tolerance for the poisonous effects of nicotine develops in a matter of hours (as compared to days or weeks for heroin and months for alcohol).

In the form of cigarettes, tobacco is one of the most addictive drugs known, equivalent to crack cocaine and ice. It is harder to break the habit of smoking cigarettes than it is to stop using heroin or alcohol. Moreover, many people learn to use alcohol and heroin in nonaddictive ways, whereas very few cigarette smokers can avoid becoming addicts. Occasionally, you will meet someone who smokes two or three cigarettes a day or even two or three a week, but such people are rare. Interestingly, these occasional users get high from smoking and like the effect, while most addicted smokers do not experience major changes in consciousness.

Smoke from cigarettes inhaled deeply delivers concentrated nicotine to vital brain centers within a few seconds — faster than heroin reaches the brain when it is injected into a vein in the arm. This probably explains why smoking cigarettes is so addictive.

Treatment of tobacco addiction is very difficult. Doctors frequently prescribe substitute forms of nicotine, such as chewing gum and skin patches, to help addicts through the physical withdrawal, but these methods often fail to curb the psychological craving for cigarettes.

Doctors know also that regular cigarette smoking is a leading cause of serious disease of the lungs, heart, and blood vessels. This does not mean that everyone who smokes will necessarily get lung cancer. Some people smoke heavily all their lives and show no ill effects, probably because they have healthy lungs and strong constitutions to begin with. Others are not so lucky.

Pipes and cigars are less hazardous than cigarettes because smoke from them is harsher, discouraging deep inhalation. Many smokers of pipes and cigars do not inhale at all and so completely avoid the risk of lung disease. In addition, since pipes and cigars don't deliver rapid pulses of nicotine to the brain, pipe and cigar smokers are less likely than cigarette smokers to become addicted to tobacco so strongly or so fast. Pipes and cigars are not without risk, however. They still put nicotine into the body, affecting the heart and circulation, and increase the risk of cancer of the lips, mouth, and throat.

Another health hazard of tobacco is secondhand smoke. If you live or work with smokers, you can inhale the equivalent of smoking one-half to one pack of cigarettes a day, raising your risk of tobacco-associated disease. (The smoke coming off the lighted end of a cigarette actually contains more toxins than smoke inhaled through the other end, which has been filtered through a mat of tobacco.)

Some tobacco users take the drug without burning it. Tobacco chewers place wads of it in their mouth, letting the nicotine diffuse into their system through blood vessels in their tongue and cheeks. Others use snuff (finely powdered tobacco) by inhaling it or putting pinches of it in their mouth. Many Amazonian Indians cook tobacco and water to form a paste that they rub on their gums.

All of these preparations provide strong stimulation in the form of high doses of nicotine — higher than cigarettes, pipes, and cigars — because burning destroys so much of the nicotine in tobacco. Nevertheless, chewing tobacco or taking snuff is less addicting than smoking because it puts nicotine into the blood and brain much less directly.

Most people who use snuff or chewing tobacco for the first time dislike it. These products burn the mouth or nose, taste terrible, cause intense salivation and sneezing, and often produce rapid dizziness and nausea. With repeated trials, however, users grow tolerant of the worst effects and come to like the sensations in their mouth and nose. Tobacco companies now sell snuff as "smokeless tobacco," some of it with mint and fruit flavoring to make it more acceptable to novices. The companies promote it as a new and pleasant way to use the drug, even in nonsmoking areas. Smokeless tobaccos have recently become popular among teen-agers, probably because it is easier to use the drug without detection. An unquestionable plus for snuff users and tobacco chewers is that they do not pollute the air with smoke and expose nonusers to nicotine and other irritants.

Despite growing awareness of its toxicity and addictiveness, tobacco remains an accepted drug in our society. Its use is even encouraged by extensive advertising that makes smokers seem mature and sexually appealing. Our government actively supports the tobacco industry with public funds. Certainly, this is an example of how our division of drugs into good and evil is not at all rational.

New World natives used tobacco in religious and magical rituals thousands of years ago, and some South American Indians still use strong tobacco as a consciousness-altering drug today. On special occasions, they build giant cigars that the men take turns inhaling. They quickly become very intoxicated. Because they do not use tobacco except on special occasions, they have no tolerance for its effects and so get very high. In North America today, all Indian medicine men and women use tobacco ceremonially; they believe that tobacco smoke carries their prayers to the spirit world. When the Spanish discovered America, they observed Indians using tobacco and began using it themselves.

In the 1500s, Europeans also used tobacco to alter consciousness. It was a scarce and precious substance from the New World, and people smoked it occasionally, inhaling as deeply as they could and holding the smoke in their lungs to maximize the effect. Early tobacco was so harsh that people could not do this often enough to develop rapid tolerance and addiction. Still, authorities at the time were very upset at what they considered to be a new form of evil and tried their best to prohibit tobacco use. In many countries, the penalty for people caught possessing tobacco was death.

Needless to say, these measures did not work, as criminal penalties for drug use never do. Tobacco supplies grew, and more people began smoking more and more regularly. As tobacco became increasingly common, it lost its special significance, and its users, instead of getting high on it once in a while, became addicts who needed it just to feel normal. Governments then began to see in tobacco a new source of revenue, which they depend on to this day. The development of milder tobaccos, which could be inhaled deeply and often, gave birth to cigarette addiction as we know it today and with it the rise of the modern tobacco industry. Throughout the first half of the twentieth century, authorities encouraged the use of tobacco on the grounds that it promoted concentration and relaxation. In movies of the 1930s and 1940s, all the characters smoke incessantly. During World War II, cigarettes were standard issue in the rations for American soldiers, and as late as the 1950s, doctors appeared in cigarette ads promoting particular brands as "soothing to the throat."

Toward the end of the twentieth century, society's views on tobacco began to change. Smoking became unfashionable as a result of persistent educational efforts, nonsmokers began to demand and get smoke-free environments, and smokers became second-class citizens. Smoking is now banned on airplanes and buses and in airports, as well as many restaurants and bars. Workplace smoking has been virtually eradicated. A large number of cities and towns have banned smoking in all public places. Norway has done it for the whole country, with other European countries considering similar legislation.

In 1998, Mississippi became the first state to instigate litigation against the four largest cigarette-producing companies (collectively known as Big Tobacco), seeking compensation for tobacco-related health care costs. Florida, Minnesota, and Texas soon followed suit. The states settled their lawsuits for a combined total of $40 billion. The remaining states and the District of Columbia later settled a major class action lawsuit against Big Tobacco for $206 billion.

There is legitimate reason for the concern about the health effects of tobacco smoking. A recent British government study of adolescents shows that a youngster who smokes more than *one* cigarette has only a 15 percent chance of remaining a nonsmoker. If you are thinking about experimenting with tobacco, especially in the form of cigarettes, consider the fact that most experimenters fall into this trap and become addicts before they know it.

Four Exotic Stimulant Plants

Betel. The betel nut is the spicy-tasting seed of a tropical palm tree. In Asia, millions of people chew it daily, combining it with a pinch of lime (the alkaline mineral, not the fruit) and wrapping it in a fresh leaf of another plant called the betel pepper. This combination produces a great deal of red juice, which betel chewers spit

out. In India, this mixture is called *pan* and is often livened up
with spices like clove and sugar and enjoyed as an after-dinner digestive aid. Betel nut contains a drug called arecoline, a stimulant
comparable to caffeine. Betel chewing is a habit that is similar to
the habits of chewing gum and drinking coffee or cola drinks in
industrialized societies. Betel juice stains teeth black over time.
Heavy use may increase the risk of oral cancers.

Qat (khat, chat, miraa). Qat is a popular stimulant in a wide area
of east Africa and the Middle East. It is a shrubby tree whose fresh
leaves and young twigs are eaten for their stimulating effect. The
leaves lose their power when they dry out. Qat contains many active chemicals, some of which resemble amphetamines in their
structure. Unlike coca, the leaves of qat, which have a bitter, as-
tringent taste, are usually swallowed. Truck drivers in Kenya are
big users of this plant. (It is called *miraa* there.) Ethiopia is a major
producing country. In fact, Ethiopian Airlines was formed to deliver fresh qat to Yemen, a country with many consumers but no
production, because it is a desert. In the United States, qat is
sometimes sold under the table at Ethiopian restaurants.

Yohimbe. Yohimbe, the bark of an African tree with a bitter, spicy
taste, contains a drug called yohimbine that is used in a few prescription medicines to treat sexual impotence in men. Yohimbe
bark is available at some herb stores and can be brewed into a
stimulating tea. It is supposed to be an aphrodisiac, and some users say that it causes tingling feelings along the spine.

Ephedra. Ephedras are leafless bushes that grow in deserts
throughout the world. They are related to pine trees and bear tiny
cones. Several species contain the drug ephedrine, a stimulant
and a remedy for asthma. American ephedra, found throughout
the western United States, is known as Mormon tea because early
Mormon settlers used it instead of caffeine beverages, which are
prohibited by their religion. Until recently, herb stores sold both

American ephedra and the much stronger Chinese type. The dry stems are boiled with water to make a pleasant-tasting tea that can be very stimulating. Chinese ephedra and ephedrine were common ingredients of herbal uppers sold in health food stores for weight loss and energy. Manufacturers have often packed these products with high doses of these herbs and added caffeine for good measure. Adverse reactions, including a few deaths, were common in people who took these products. Sensational publicity about the dangers of ephedra and ephedrine prompted Congress to ban them in 2004. Ephedra will still be allowed in Chinese herbal medical formulas.

Over-the-Counter (OTC) Drugs

Many cold remedies and other over-the-counter preparations contain caffeine to offset the drowsiness caused by antihistamines. (See pages 173–75 for a description of the effects of antihistamines.) Another stimulant in these products is pseudoephedrine, used as a nasal decongestant. Also look for synephrine, sometimes concealed as "bitter orange extract."

Some Rules for Using Stimulants Safely

Because stimulants are so common, most people will use one or another at some time. If you become involved with stimulants, here are some rules that will help you stay in a good relationship with them.

1. *Limit* your *frequency of use.* All trouble with stimulants arises from using them too often. If you like the feeling a stimulant gives, it is all too easy to let your frequency of use creep up. Set limits! For example, never take a stimulant two days in a row.
2. *Use stimulants purposefully.* Taking these drugs just to feel good will not help you limit your use. If you are going to take a stimulant, you should use the stimulation for something — a physical or mental task, for instance. One side benefit of such

purposeful use is that the satisfaction of accomplishment will
offset the letdown when the drug wears off.

3. *Do not take stimulants to help you perform ordinary functions.*
You should be able to get up in the morning, move your bowels, and make it through the afternoon without drugs. If you
cannot, you should change your patterns of diet, sleep, and exercise. Relying on stimulants for everyday activity leads to too-
frequent use and dependence.

4. *Take stimulants by mouth.* Putting these drugs more directly
into the bloodstream (as by snorting, smoking, or shooting)
accentuates the letdown that follows the high and encourages
frequent administration. It also increases the harmful effects
on the body.

5. *Take dilute forms of stimulants rather than concentrated ones.* The
more dilute the preparation of a stimulant, the easier it is for
the body to adjust to it and the more gentle the letdown at the
end. Preparations of plants such as coffee and tea are naturally more dilute than refined or synthetic drugs and are easier to stay in good relationships with.

6. *Maintain good habits of nutrition, rest, and exercise.* Remember
that stimulants force your body to give up its stores of chemical energy. Whenever you use stimulants, especially if you
take them with any regularity, it is important to let your body
recharge itself. The healthier you are, the less you will feel that
you need outside stimulation.

7. *Do not combine stimulants with depressants or other drugs.* Combinations of drugs always complicate matters. Some people
can't sleep at night because they take too many stimulants
during the day. So they take depressants at night. Then they
can't get moving in the morning and have to take more stimulants. This pattern of drug-taking quickly leads to trouble.

8. *Avoid look-alike drugs.* They have nothing to recommend them.

It should not be difficult to use stimulants wisely and stay in
good relationships with them. They are not the answer to the ups

and downs of life, and taking them to try to avoid the downs only leads to problems. Nor do they give anything for nothing. Users pay later for any energy and good feeling that stimulants give them. If you remain aware of what stimulants are and how they work, you will be able to avoid the trap of becoming dependent on them.

SUGGESTED READING

Coffee and tea are the subjects of *The Book of Coffee and Tea* by Meri Shardin (second revised edition; New York: St. Martin's Press, 1996). A classic book on the colorful history of coffee and human beings is *Coffee: The Epic of a Commodity* by Heinrich Eduard Jacob and Kynn Alley (Springfield, N.J.: Burford Books, 1999). The most famous work on tea is Kakuzo Okakura's *The Book of Tea* (Boston: Charles E. Tuttle, 1956), first published in 1906. About much more than tea, it is an elegant treatise on Japanese culture and philosophy written to help dispel Western misconceptions about Japan. A more recent work on the same subject is *Tea: The Eyelids of Bodhidhaima* by Eelco Hesse (Berkeley, Calif.: And/Or Press, 1982). An interesting book on the origins and development of Coca-Cola is *For God, Country, and Coca-Cola: The Definitive History of the Great American Soft Drink and the Company That Makes It* by Mark Pendergrast (second edition; New York: Basic Books, 2000). Chocolate devotees may be interested in a book by Sandra Boynton called *Chocolate: The Consuming Passion* (New York: Workman, 1982), a profile and ardent defense of that substance by a self-proclaimed chocoholic. See also Allen M. Young's *The Chocolate Tree: A Natural History of Cacao* (Washington, D.C.: Smithsonian Institution Press, 1994), a detailed examination of the source of chocolate.

Many books on coca and cocaine are available. Here is a selection of the best:

W. Golden Mortimer's *History of Coca: Divine Plant of the Incas* (Corvallis, Oreg.: University Press of the Pacific, 2000) was first published in 1901. It is a long description of Incan civilization, Peru, and coca and contains valuable information. An excellent book on the origins and history of cocaine is *Cocaine: Global Histories,* edited by Paul Gootenberg (New York: Routledge, 1999). Dominic Streatfield's *Co-*

caine: An Unauthorized Biography (New York: Picador USA, 2003) is a well-researched, humorous narrative on the subject, with accounts of the author's visits to crack houses, maximum security prisons, and the South American rain forest. In *Cocaine: From Medical Marvel to Modern Menace in the United States, 1884–1920* (Baltimore: Johns Hopkins University Press, 2000), Joseph F. Spillane investigates lesser-known facets of the drug's history, including the role of American business in helping to create interest in it.

For firsthand accounts of cocaine abuse, see *Cocaine Changes: The Experience of Using and Quitting* by Dan Waldorf (Philadelphia: Temple University Press, 1991). The book includes over two hundred interviews with heavy cocaine users and concludes that the national hysteria over the drug is largely unfounded. The horrors of crack houses are recounted in *Crackhouse: Notes from the End of the Line* (New York: Perseus, 1992) by Terry Williams and Terence T. Williams. *The Seven Per Cent Solution* by Nicholas Meyer (New York: Dutton, 1974) is a novel that concerns Sherlock Holmes's cocaine habit. It was made into a popular movie. The problems and perils of freebasing cocaine are brilliantly depicted by comedian Richard Pryor in his movie *Richard Pryor: Live on the Sunset Strip*. Pryor's real-life habit of freebasing cocaine resulted in a near-fatal accident. An excellent movie about the cocaine trade is *Blow*.

Despite their widespread use, amphetamines have attracted far less attention from writers than cocaine. All of the best books are out of print. The best of all, *Synthetic Panics: The Symbolic Politics of Designer Drugs* by Philip Jenkins (New York: New York University Press, 1999), is readily available on the Internet. For a firsthand account of methamphetamine abuse, see *Meth= Sorcery: Know the Truth* by Steve Box (Above All Distributing, 2000).

Recent years have finally seen the appearance of a few good books on tobacco. *Regulating Tobacco: Premises and Policy Options* (New York: Oxford University Press, 2001), edited by Robert L. Rabin and Stephen D. Sugarman, is an excellent collection of essays on strategies that have influenced tobacco use. An interesting and surprising account of the antismoking movement is *For Your Own Good: The Anti-Smoking Crusade and the Tyranny of Public Health* by Jay S. Cohen (New York: Tarcher/Putnam, 2001). John Barth's novel *The Sot-Weed Factor* (New

York: Bantam, 1969) revolves around tobacco. Probably, the best account of cigarette addiction occurs in a comic novel by Italo Svevo, *Further Confessions of Zeno* (Berkeley: University of California Press, 1969). The author describes the endless tricks and self-deceptions used by a cigarette addict, as well as the low probability of cure.

The best book available on qat is John G. Kennedy's *The Flower of Paradise: The Institutionalized Use of the Drug Qat in North Yemen* (Boston: D. Reidel, 1987).

7. Depressants

DEPRESSANTS ARE DRUGS that lower the energy level of the nervous system, reducing sensitivity to outside stimulation and, in high doses, inducing sleep. Many depressants are used medically and socially, and many are consumed illegally. In fact, depressants include some of the most popular drugs that affect mood.

At first glance, it may seem odd that people would want to take substances in order to depress their nervous systems. Who wants to feel groggy and depressed? Actually, depressants make people sleepy and stuporous only in high doses; in lower doses, they often make people relaxed and happy. Alcohol is a good example. One or two drinks can make people feel cheerful, alert, and more alive, while three or four can make them drunk, with obvious symptoms of reduced brain function.

Scientists don't really know why low doses of depressants make people feel stimulated. One theory is that the first parts of the brain to be depressed are inhibitory centers that normally act to dampen mood. As the dose is increased, more and more parts of the nervous system are slowed down. Very high doses of depressants can cause coma, in which all consciousness is lost; a person in a coma is insensible to all stimulation — even loud noise and intense pain. Still higher doses of these drugs can shut down the most vital centers in the brain, such as the one that controls respiration, resulting in a quick death from lack of oxygen.

Depressant drugs are more dangerous than stimulants because overdoses of depressants are apt to kill people by interfering with vital brain centers. Also, depressants produce a wider variety of effects, from relaxation and euphoria in low doses to unresponsive coma in very high doses.

Depressants include several distinct categories of drugs, each with its own benefits and dangers.

Sedative-Hypnotics

This large category of depressants comprises alcohol, "sleeping pills," and antianxiety drugs. In low doses, these drugs promote relaxation and restfulness (sedation), especially in the daytime. Larger doses, especially at night, induce sleep (the word *hypnosis* comes from the name of the Greek god of sleep). The term *sedative-hypnotic* refers to this double action.

Alcohol (Ethyl Alcohol, Ethanol)

Alcohol is the most popular psychoactive drug in the world, used every day by many millions of people. Probably, it is also the oldest drug known to human beings, because it is easy to discover that fruits and juices, left to stand in a warm place, soon ferment into an alcoholic mixture. Alcohol is so commonplace and its effects, both good and bad, are so well known that they need little description. Anyone who has felt the pleasant stimulation of a glass of wine knows the beneficial side of this drug. Anyone who has interacted with a drunk person knows how powerful and unpleasant alcohol can be in overdose. Anyone who has lived with an alcoholic can attest to the horrors of alcohol addiction.

Production of ethyl alcohol depends upon yeast, which feeds on sugar, making alcohol and carbon dioxide as by-products. Yeasts are simple one-celled forms of life found everywhere — in the air and on the skins of many fruits, especially grapes. To grow and multiply, yeast cells need water, sugar, and warmth. They keep on growing until they use up all the sugar or until the rising concentration of alcohol kills them. Alcohol is a poison as well as a drug; in high enough doses, it kills living things, including the yeasts that make it.

Natural sources of sugar available to primitive people were fruit and honey, both of which can be made into wine with a maximum alcohol content of about 12 percent. Starch is also a potential source of alcohol, but enzymes must convert starch to sugar before yeast can digest it. There are enzymes in saliva that can accomplish this, and one of the earliest kinds of beer was made by natives in tropical America who learned to chew corn to a pulp, spit it into clay pots, mix it with water, and let it ferment. Sprouting grains also produce usable enzymes; in standard beer making, sprouted barley (malt) is used to convert the starch of grains to sugar so that yeast can grow and produce alcohol. The alcohol content of beer is usually less than half that of wine. Beer is also more nutritious than wine because it has a lot of calories in the form of carbohydrates.

Distilled alcohol is a relatively new product, only a few hundred years old: brandy was the first distilled liquor made; it was obtained by heating wine and then cooling and condensing the vapors in another container. This process increases the alcohol content dramatically: from 12 percent up to 40 or 50 percent. The original idea of distillers was to concentrate wine so that its volume would be smaller, to make it easier to ship it in barrels overseas. At the end of the voyage, the brandy was to be diluted with water for an alcohol content of 12 percent. What happened, of course, was that when people got their hands on what was in the barrels, no one waited to add water. Suddenly, a new and powerful form of alcohol flooded the world.

Our society now manufactures and consumes many distilled liquors. Scotch and bourbon whiskeys are made from beerlike preparations of grain. Rum is distilled from fermented molasses; vodka is just diluted ethyl alcohol (so is gin, with flavor added), also usually distilled from grain. Because of their much higher alcohol content, these hard liquors are stronger and more intoxicating than fermented drinks.

From earliest times, people probably used beer and wine much as we use them today: as social and recreational drugs, to dispel

I like alcohol. It is a powerful drug and, God knows, for some people a hellish one, but if used carefully it can give great pleasure. After a long, hard day, the splendid warm glow that strong drink provides is one of my favorite feelings; it starts in the pit of my stomach, then spreads to my limbs and brain. I know that alcohol is a depressant, but it acts and feels like a gentle relaxant — of the spirit as well as of the physical body. Just notice the increased vivacity and noise level at a cocktail party after a drink has been served to see how alcohol can put people at ease emotionally.

— sixty-two-year-old man, psychoanalyst

worry and anxiety, to feel high, and as a change from the dull routines of work. Our early ancestors probably also noticed that the effects of alcohol were variable and related to the dose, and that some people became dependent on alcohol.

Alcohol is absorbed very quickly from the digestive system, enters the bloodstream, and reaches the brain, where it causes its effects on mood and behavior. The body has to work hard to eliminate alcohol; it burns some of it as fuel and excretes some unchanged in the breath and urine. The burden of metabolizing alcohol falls especially on the liver.

The effects of alcohol are directly related to how much of it is in the blood at any time. Low concentrations, particularly at the beginning of drinking, cause alertness, a good mood, feelings of energy, warmth, and confidence, and the dissipation of anxiety and inhibition. Most people find these changes pleasant.

It is important to note, however, that some of the sensations produced by low doses of alcohol — especially the sense of confidence — may be false. Unlike stimulants, alcohol and other depressants slow the functioning of the nervous system, including reflexes, reaction time, and efficiency of muscular response. Although people often feel that they are performing better after a few drinks, scientific tests show otherwise. This is one source of danger in using depressant drugs to feel good: the false sense of confidence can lead people to take unwarranted risks, such as driving a car while the imbiber is in a condition that favors disaster.

Similarly, the sense of warmth produced by drinking is deceptive. It is due to increased blood flow to the skin, which allows more heat to radiate to the outside of the body. In fact, inner body temperature is dropping even as the sensation of warmth increases, so that people who dress inadequately for cold weather and drink in order to feel warm may fall victim to hypothermia.

Another example of the deceptive nature of alcohol is its sexual effect. Many people who drink to enhance sex claim that alcohol increases desire, removes inhibitions, and promotes relaxation. In men, however, the depression of the nervous system by alcohol can prevent erection and drastically interfere with sexual performance. Writers as far back as Shakespeare have noted this property of alcohol. In act 2, scene 3, of *Macbeth*, the following exchange occurs between Macduff and a porter in Macbeth's castle:

MACDUFF: What three things does drink especially provoke?
PORTER: Marry, sir, nose painting, sleep, and urine. Lechery, sir, it provokes, and unprovokes; it provokes the desire, but it takes away the performance.

People who drink should be aware that their subjective impressions while under the influence of alcohol may not correspond to reality.

Further, it is clear that, as with any psychoactive drug, the pleasant feelings that alcohol can provide depend as much on set and setting as on pharmacological action. The same amount of wine that makes someone pleasantly high at a party may make a depressed person in a lonely room even more depressed.

The concentration of alcohol in the bloodstream is determined by several factors: first, by the concentration of alcohol in the drink; second, by the rate of drinking; third, by the presence or absence of food in the stomach; and fourth, by the rate at which the body can metabolize and eliminate alcohol.

The stronger the drink, the faster the blood alcohol level will rise and the sooner a person will get drunk. Gulping down cocktails and drinking wine like water are good ways to speed through the more pleasant, early effects of alcohol intoxication and go right to the less desirable ones.

Food in the stomach, especially milk, slows down absorption of alcohol into the blood. Therefore, drinking on an empty stomach can result in faster and more intense drunkenness. Eating before and during drinking moderates the intensity of alcohol's effects.

Finally, some people metabolize alcohol more rapidly than others and so can handle larger doses. This may be genetically determined; if so, some people could inherit a tendency to become alcoholic. People who drink alcohol regularly metabolize it faster than people who do not, and regular drinkers won't be affected by doses that nondrinkers would certainly feel. This is tolerance, and it develops quickly for alcohol and other sedative-hypnotics. Alcoholics show very high tolerance for the drug; they can even survive doses of alcohol that would kill nondrinkers. Other people may have lower than normal abilities to metabolize alcohol. Some Japanese, for example, have an inborn biochemical quirk that causes them to get drunk on doses of wine or liquor that would hardly affect most Americans or Europeans.

As alcohol increases in the bloodstream, it depresses more and more of the nervous system, producing the familiar symptoms of drunkenness: slurred speech, incoordination, insensitivity to pain, and inappropriate behavior. People become drunk in very different ways, depending on their personalities, their mood at the time, and the social setting. Some people become boisterous and obnoxious; others become overly friendly, confiding the most intimate details of their lives to perfect strangers. Some people get belligerent, even violent, while others become gloomy, tearful, and self-pitying.

Drunkenness is a serious problem throughout the world, accounting for many accidents, acts of violence, injuries, and deaths. Many traffic accidents are directly related to alcohol intoxication, as are many murders. It isn't uncommon for drunk people to kill friends or relatives and have no memory of these events the next day, a consequence of alcohol's depressant effect on parts of the brain responsible for reason, thought, and memory.

Most people who get drunk eventually fall into stuporous sleep. When they wake up, they are hung over, with such symptoms as sour stomach, headache, weakness, shakiness, depression, and inability to concentrate, work, or think clearly. These symptoms reflect the toxic effects of alcohol on the body and are very uncomfortable. Alcohol is strongly diuretic — that is, it increases the flow of urine, causing the body to lose water. A night of hard drinking can result in serious dehydration if the drinker does not replace the lost water, and this condition may contribute to the discomfort of the next day's hangover.

Because additional alcohol ("the hair of the dog that bit you") makes a hung-over person feel better in the short run, excessive drinking can lead to further drinking and start people on the path to dependence.

Dependence on alcohol is a true addiction, marked by extreme craving for the drug, tolerance, and withdrawal. The craving for alcohol among alcoholics is legendary and has been the subject of many books and films (see pages 107–108). Recovering alcoholics tell frightening stories of the lengths to which they went to obtain their drug when deprived and of squandering all of their money on drink. Withdrawal from alcohol is a major medical crisis. Some of its worst forms, such as delirium tremens (the DTs), can be fatal and are more serious than withdrawal from narcotics.

Moreover, because alcohol is such a strong and toxic drug, prolonged regular use can cause tremendous physical damage. Cirrhosis of the liver, in which normal liver cells are replaced by use-less scar tissue, is a direct and common result of overuse of alcohol and leads to many distressing symptoms, among them, loss of sexual potency and inability to digest food. The other or-gans that bear the brunt of alcohol's poisonous effect are the brain and the peripheral nervous system. Alcoholics develop shakes, amnesia, and loss of intellect, which may reflect permanent dam-age to nerves. The list of medical problems associated with exces-sive drinking is much too long to reproduce here. It includes ad-verse effects on unborn babies of alcoholic women (fetal alcohol syndrome) and increased susceptibility to such infectious diseases as pneumonia and tuberculosis. Hospitals around the world are filled with chronic medical patients whose bodies are ravaged by alcohol.

Alcoholism is also one of the most stubborn forms of drug ad-diction, very resistant to treatment. Many doctors who work with alcoholics admit that they have little success with them. The only groups that seem to be able to help are Alcoholics Anonymous, which depends on an almost religious adherence to a group ethic, and the Native American Church, which uses peyote in religious rituals and vigorously crusades against drinking among American Indians (see pages 123–24).

Not all regular drinkers become alcoholics. In fact, most regular drinkers are not addicted. Some people may inherit a tendency to become addicted because of peculiarities in their biochemistry or metabolism. Children of alcoholics are more likely to grow up to be alcoholics, but so are the children of two teetotalers. That sug-gests that a childhood lack of good role models for healthy drink-ing may also be an important factor.

One of the clearest signs of alcoholism is repeated drinking to get drunk. Alcoholics cannot limit their intake to a social drink or two; they invariably go much further. But drunkenness isn't much fun, either at the time or the following day. Why, then, do so many people consume overdoses of alcohol?

> Although I kept trying to use alcohol moderately, whenever I'd set out to get high on it, I would always keep on drinking till I got drunk, no matter how many resolutions I made not to . . . I've tried various drugs since those days and don't think anything comes close to alcohol in terms of raw strength and potential for trouble. I couldn't learn to control it well, and I see many people around me who have the same problem.
>
> — thirty-seven-year-old man, college professor

This question points up the main problem with alcohol. As noted earlier, most people like the early effects of the drug, which resemble those of stimulants, but taking more of it dramatically changes the quality of the effects. It isn't easy for people to learn how to stay within the dose range that makes them feel good; it is very easy to cross into the zone of unpleasant effects and regret it. Young people beginning to drink should recognize that this is a problem that they will have to deal with by acquiring experience. Many people — if they are metabolically normal, come from supportive families, and don't have serious psychological problems — learn how to control their intake of alcohol and keep from sliding into the trouble zone, but others do not.

Alcohol is one of the most difficult drugs to control because it is so strong and because the dose-related difference in its effects is so great. Used intelligently, alcohol can relieve stress. Some people even claim that alcohol promotes health. For example, some medical studies suggest that moderate drinking decreases the risk of heart attacks by reducing the clotting tendency of the blood and by improving the metabolizing of cholesterol. Wine lovers say that drinking wine with meals aids digestion. Some physicians think that old people benefit from alcohol in small amounts. These claims may be true. Unfortunately, some people cannot learn to drink moderately. Recovering alcoholics, for example, usually become drunks again very quickly if they try to drink socially.

There is no question that alcohol is the most toxic of all the drugs discussed in this book. Yet our own society has made alcohol its social drug of choice. It is widely available in many attractive forms, extensively advertised, and used to the point that it is hard to avoid. In certain groups, liquor is so much the required social lubricant that nondrinkers feel uncomfortable and out of place. Alcohol comes into people's lives at every turn. Friends give each other bottles of liquor as holiday gifts. Airlines sell drinks in flight and placate passengers with free drinks if planes are delayed unduly. Billboards and magazines everywhere extol the pleasures of drinking. Everyone in our society must learn to come to terms with this powerful drug.

Unless you are a Muslim or a Mormon or belong to some other group that prohibits its use altogether, you will have to learn how to refuse alcohol if you don't want to drink or how to drink it intelligently and not let your use get out of control.

Some Suggestions for Using Alcohol Wisely

1. Define what benefits you want from alcohol. Remember that alcohol is attractive because it can make people feel temporarily better, both physically and mentally. You can enjoy these good effects if you learn to use the drug carefully and purposefully. If you feel feverish and achy from flu, going to bed and taking a small drink may be a good remedy. If you walk into a party and feel awkward, anxious, and inhibited, a little alcohol may help you get into the swing of things.

2. It is good to make rules about when and where *not* to drink. For example, a person who uses alcohol to relax after a hard day shouldn't drink at the end of an easy one or before a day is done. No one should drink and drive.

3. Rules about times, places, and situations that are appropriate

for drinking help control the tendency of alcohol to get out of hand. You might decide to drink with friends but not by yourself, on weekends and holidays but not during the week, after sunset but not during the day.

4. Learn to regulate the amount of alcohol in your bloodstream. Once it's there, only time can get it out. You can control the rate of absorption of alcohol into your blood by drinking dilute forms of it rather than concentrated ones (for example, by adding water to wine and mixers to hard liquor). You can also make sure that you have food in your stomach before and during drinking. You can practice consuming alcoholic drinks slowly. Finally, you can practice saying no to more drinks when you've had enough.

5. Whenever you consume alcohol heavily, remember to drink plenty of plain water to offset fluid losses from increased urination. By doing so, you may moderate the next day's hangover.

6. Don't spend time with people who drink to excess or encourage you to drink more than you want.

7. Be careful about falling into patterns of regular drinking to deal with ongoing emotional problems, such as anxiety or depression. Alcohol may mask the symptoms temporarily, but it cannot solve the problems, and this kind of use is more likely to lead to dependence.

8. Adolescence, with its confusions, peer pressures, and tendency toward rebellion, is a time when unhealthy patterns of drug use can develop that may persist into later life and be very hard to break. Young people may think that they aren't as susceptible to dependence on alcohol as adults, but the evidence contradicts this view. Alcohol is a difficult drug to control at any age, and alcoholism doesn't appear overnight. It is the result of unwise drinking over time, beginning with the earliest experience with the drug.

9. Alcohol contains calories. If you are trying to lose weight, watch your intake.

10. The best way to protect yourself from the harmful effects of al-
    cohol is not to drink it every day.
11. If you drink regularly, make sure that you maintain good hab-
    its of rest, exercise, and nutrition. In particular, take supple-
    mental vitamin B-1 (thiamine), 100 milligrams a day on days
    that you drink. Alcohol selectively destroys this vitamin. Also,
    take milk thistle, a nontoxic herb that protects liver cells from
    chemical damage.
12. If you begin to suspect that you have problems with drinking,
    or if people who know you think that you do, seek help from
    professionals. It is difficult or impossible to deal with problem
    drinking without outside help.

Barbiturates and Other Sleeping Pills ("Downers")

This class of sedative-hypnotic drugs — loosely known as sleeping pills, or downers — has been around for some time. They are
manufactured both legally and illegally and are widely used. Medical doctors prescribe these substances in low doses to calm people
during the day and in higher doses to help them sleep at night.
There are millions of people who take sleeping pills every night
and can't fall asleep without them. Millions of others take downers
for nonmedical reasons: to get high, to feel good, or to party.

Barbituric acid was discovered in 1864. Since then, a number of
derivatives of it have been introduced. They are all known as barbiturates and are the most important drugs in this class. The first
barbiturate sleeping drug, called barbital, appeared in 1903. The
second, called phenobarbital, appeared in 1912. Hundreds of barbiturates are now known, and many are in use today.

Some of the barbiturates are slowly metabolized and eliminated
by the kidneys. Barbital and phenobarbital are in this group and
are known as long-acting barbiturates because their effects last
twelve to twenty-four hours. They are used as daytime sedatives
more than as nighttime hypnotics, and since they don't produce
much euphoria or stimulation, few people take them to get high.

Another group of barbiturates is more rapidly metabolized by the liver. Their effects last six or seven hours, and they are called short acting. They include amobarbital (Amytal), pentobarbital (Nembutal), hexobarbital (Sombulex), and secobarbital (Seconal). These drugs behave very much like alcohol, giving pleasant feelings in low doses, especially as they begin to take effect. Therefore, some people seek them out to change the way they feel, and there is no shortage of these drugs on the black market.

Finally, there are very short-acting barbiturates that produce almost immediate unconsciousness when injected intravenously. Thiopental (Pentothal) is the main example; dentists and doctors use it as an anesthetic for surgical operations. Since it wipes out awareness quickly and leaves no memory of the experience, no one takes it for fun.

When people talk about taking downers, they usually mean the short-acting barbiturates or a few similar drugs that we will discuss later. All of these substances are like alcohol, and most of the statements in the alcohol section apply to downers as well (see pages 72–78). Sleeping pills can make people feel and look drunk, leave users with hangovers, kill when taken in overdose by knocking out the respiratory center of the brain, and produce stubborn addiction with dangerous withdrawal syndromes, marked in some cases by convulsions and death.

Since the similarities between downers and alcohol are so numerous, it might be easier to talk about how they differ.

Unlike alcohol, sleeping pills are noncaloric; the body cannot burn them as fuel but must metabolize them in other ways. They are also not as toxic as alcohol over time and don't cause the kind of liver disease and other medical damage so common in alcoholics. Tolerance for downers occurs, as with alcohol, but there is an important and curious difference. As people use downers regularly, tolerance for the effects on mood develops faster than tolerance for the lethal dose. For this reason, people run a greater risk of accidentally killing themselves with downers. For example, people who get into the habit of taking sleeping pills every night to fall asleep might start out with one a night, progress to two, then

> The barbiturate addict presents a shocking spectacle. He cannot coordinate, he staggers, falls off bar stools, goes to sleep in the middle of a sentence, drops food out of his mouth. He is confused, quarrelsome, and stupid. And he almost always uses other drugs, anything he can lay his hands on: alcohol, benzedrine, opiates, marijuana. Barbiturate users are looked down on in addict society: "Goof-ball bums. They got no class to them." . . . It seems to me that barbiturates cause the worst possible form of addiction, unsightly, deteriorating, difficult to treat.
>
> — **William S. Burroughs, from his novel *Naked Lunch* (1959)**

graduate to four to get the same effect. One night the dose that they need to fall asleep might also be the dose that stops their breathing.

Because their depressant effects are additive, combining alcohol and downers is especially dangerous. A dose of alcohol that a person is used to, combined with a dose of a downer that would be all right by itself, may lead to coma and death. Many people have died because they were ignorant of this fact.

As with alcohol, the effects of downers on mood are extremely variable, depending on individual personality, expectation, and setting. Some people who take sleeping pills feel nothing but sleepiness. Others fight off the sleepiness and say that they feel high. A dose of Seconal taken at a wild party might inspire violent excitement, whereas a person taking the same dose in a quiet room might be overcome with lethargy. Some medical patients have strange reactions to prescribed downers, becoming anxious and agitated instead of calm. Old people are likely to become intoxicated on ordinary doses, as are people with liver or kidney disease.

Most people take these drugs by mouth, but injectable forms are available. In hospitals, hypnotic doses of Nembutal are often given by intramuscular injection, especially to patients who cannot take medicine by mouth. On the street, some users inject barbiturates intravenously (sometimes crushing and dissolving oral preparations), a practice that greatly increases their toxicity.

Other users like to combine downers and stimulants, claiming that the combined effect is more pleasant than either drug by itself. A few such combinations are even made legally for medical use. One example, Dexamyl, is a mixture of amobarbital and dextroamphetamine (Dexedrine). Supposedly, the barbiturate counteracts any tendency of the amphetamine to cause anxiety or jitteriness, while the amphetamine reinforces the potential of the barbiturate to produce euphoria. Similarly, people who use a lot of cocaine say that drinking alcohol at the same time reduces the unpleasant side effects of that drug, while the cocaine keeps them from getting drunk and minimizes hangovers. Although these combinations probably do no harm when used occasionally, they may have a higher potential for abuse than their components would if used separately, because their combination makes it easier to take larger quantities of the drugs.

Dependence on barbiturates can occur in both medical patients and street users. Doctors write vast numbers of prescriptions for sleeping pills, and many people fall into the habit of taking them every night. Certainly, it is appropriate to take these drugs when insomnia is temporary and due to a specific, identifiable cause. For instance, the death of a close friend or relative, the breakup of a family, the loss of a job, or even moving may produce serious disturbances of sleep, and sleeping pills may help during the crisis. Some people take these drugs to help them sleep on long plane flights, during other kinds of travel, after periods of intense work or stress, and when working shifts. There is no harm in taking sleeping pills a few nights in a row in such situations.

Problems arise when people take them every night over a long time. Persistent insomnia is always a symptom of other trouble, either physical or emotional. Sleeping pills treat only the symptom. Moreover, the sleep induced by downers is not the same as

> There is no question that Quaalude can be dangerous
> when used irresponsibly or that it can be addicting. As a
> recreational drug, taken on occasion in a responsible man-
> ner, it seems to me safe and interesting and gives me an
> experience different from anything else.
>
> — thirty-six-year-old man, drug counselor

natural sleep. It doesn't provide as much dreaming time, for one
thing, and is likely to be followed by a hangover. Because drug-induced sleep may not supply all the needs of body and mind, over
time it may aggravate an underlying problem. Although many
people take sleeping pills regularly for years without having to increase the dose or suffering any obvious difficulties, this kind of
usage is a form of drug dependence.

Taking downers as a means of dealing with feelings of depression or low self-esteem is probably the riskiest way of using them.
Like alcohol, these drugs may mask the symptoms temporarily,
but over time they often increase anxiety and depression, encouraging further drug-taking in a downward spiral that can end in
suicide.

As we noted earlier, there are a number of nonbarbiturate downers, the most popular of which once was methaqualone, marketed
under such brand names as Quaalude, Sopor, and Mandrax. Its effects are equivalent to those of the barbiturates, although on its
own it is less likely to depress the respiratory center in overdose.
Still, deaths have occurred as a result of combining alcohol and
methaqualone. Street users talk about "luding out" — that is, taking Quaaludes and wine to produce a numb, euphoric state.
Quaalude has gained a street reputation as a sex enhancer and
party drug. Like all downers, it can lower inhibitions and reduce
anxiety in the same way as alcohol. But also like alcohol, it will interfere with sexual performance in males and may make it more

difficult for women to experience orgasm. Real Quaalude is seldom available today, but look-alike tablets containing no methaqualone are commonly sold to gullible buyers on the black market.

Another downer, chloral hydrate, is the oldest sleeping drug still
in medical use. Although rare today, abuse of it was not uncommon
in the last century. Slipped into alcoholic drinks, it was the notorious "Mickey Finn," or "knockout drops," used to drug unsuspecting people into unconsciousness in order to rob or kidnap them.

Still other nonbarbiturate downers include glutethimide
(Doriden), methyprylon (Noludar), ethchlorvynol (Placidyl), and
paraldehyde. All of these drugs are used in medicine as hypnotics.
They sometimes find their way to the black market, where users
of illegal downers buy them. The benefits and dangers of these
downers are the same as those of the barbiturates.

The most popular downer today is zolpidem (Ambien), widely
prescribed as a sleeping pill and chemically different from the
other drugs discussed here. Its manufacturer advertises it aggres-
sively as safe and effective for regular use, but we think that it has
all the drawbacks of other downers. It is addictive, does not reproduce natural sleep, and can be abused. (Users crush and snort the
pills or cook them for injection.)

Suggestions for Using Downers Safely

1. Take sleeping pills by mouth in doses no higher than those
   recommended by doctors, pharmacists, or manufacturers.
   (Often, lower doses will do.)
2. Don't drive or operate machinery while under the influence of
   these drugs. Like alcohol, they impair judgment, coordination, and reflexes.
3. Exercise extreme caution about using downers in combination with alcohol or other depressant drugs.
4. Don't fall into the habit of relying on downers for sleep. Insomnia can usually be overcome by improving health; getting
   more exercise; cutting down on intake of stimulants, includ-

ing caffeine and tobacco; taking warm baths before bed; and
by many other means not involving drugs.

5. Be wary of relying on these drugs to get you out of bad moods.
6. Don't take downers regularly in combination with stimulants.
7. Don't take downers if you are ill, especially if you have any
   liver or kidney problems, unless they are prescribed for you by
   a doctor who is aware of your medical problems.
8. If you find yourself becoming dependent on downers, with
   tolerance or the development of any unusual physical or mental symptoms, seek professional help.

Antianxiety Drugs

The third and last class of sedative-hypnotics consists of relatively new drugs, products of the modern pharmaceutical industry.
Dating only to the mid-1950s, these drugs used to be called minor
tranquilizers, terminology that is misleading. The word *minor* was
supposed to distinguish these drugs from the "major" tranquilizers — compounds such as chlorpromazine (Thorazine), which is
used to manage psychotic patients (see pages 170–71). Actually,
these two kinds of tranquilizers are chemically and pharmacologi-
cally unrelated. Minor tranquilizers are not, as their name implies, mild drugs. There is nothing minor about their effects, the
problems that they can cause, or their potential for abuse. Since
their invention, the minor tranquilizers have achieved enormous
popularity in medicine. Doctors have written millions upon millions of prescriptions for them, and pharmaceutical companies
have made billions of dollars by promoting and selling them as
antianxiety agents. In fact, these drugs have been among the most
widely prescribed drugs in the world.

The first minor tranquilizer to be released to the world was
meprobamate; it appeared in 1954 under the brand name Miltown
(it was also marketed later as Equanil), and soon after its appearance, people were holding Miltown parties — taking the drug socially and recreationally, just to get high.

The most popular minor tranquilizers appeared in the 1960s

— a family of drugs called benzodiazepines. Some of the most famous are chlordiazepoxide (Librium), diazepam (Valium), triazolam (Halcion), alprazolam (Xanax), lorazepam (Ativan), temazepam (Restoril), and clonazepam (Klonopin). The manufacturer of Librium and Valium, once a small company selling vitamins and antacids, became one of the most powerful pharmaceutical corporations in the world.

The pharmaceutical industry has tried hard to convince doctors and patients that these chemicals are revolutionary drugs that specifically reduce anxiety, making people calm and relaxed. In fact, the benzodiazepines are just another variation on the theme of alcohol and other sedative-hypnotics, with the same tendency to produce adverse effects and dependence.

Compared with barbiturates, antianxiety drugs are safer in overdose and somewhat less dangerous in combination with alcohol. Also, the benzodiazepines are useful in relaxing tense muscles. As daytime sedatives, they produce less drowsiness than barbiturates, but they can still make driving dangerous and interfere with other motor skills, as well as with memory and clear thinking. As nighttime hypnotics, they induce sleep and may be preferable to barbiturates if anxiety or muscle tension is present or if the patient needs a sleeping pill for more than a few nights in a row. Again, however, they do not reproduce natural sleep.

Street users of benzodiazepines take them for the same reasons that they take illegal downers: to improve mood, reduce anxiety and inhibitions, and promote social interaction.

Abuse of the minor tranquilizers, particularly of Miltown, Librium, and Valium, began in the 1950s and was the direct result of irresponsible marketing and prescribing practices. In promoting these drugs, the manufacturers portrayed stresses of everyday life as diseases. For example, ads in medical journals recommended Librium for the college student whose "newly stimulated intellectual curiosity may make her more sensitive to and apprehensive about unstable national and world conditions" (in other words, if the news freaks you out, pop a Librium). Other ads suggested giving tranquilizers to harried mothers and bored housewives, to "the woman who can't get along with her new daughter-in-law," and to "the newcomer in town who can't make friends."

Critics of this kind of salesmanship pointed out that women were targets far more often than men. Just as pharmaceutical companies encouraged doctors to prescribe amphetamines to depressed housewives in the 1960s, they have urged doctors to give benzodiazepines to anxious women. Increasing opposition to these practices has curtailed them to some extent.

A newer drug of this class deserves special comment. Flunitrazepam (Rohypnol) is not approved in the United States but is marketed in the rest of the world as a remedy for insomnia and as a pre-anesthetic medication for patients undergoing surgery. It is much more potent than Valium, lasts longer (eight hours or more), and has become widely available on the black market under the name "roofies." Most users take it with other drugs. For example, they use it to enhance the high of low-quality heroin or to come down off crack cocaine. Most often, people mix it with alcohol, a potentially dangerous combination that can cause disorientation, amnesia, respiratory depression, and death. Rohypnol has gained notoriety as a "date rape" drug, when women unknowingly consume alcoholic beverages spiked with it. Some wake up naked in unfamiliar surroundings with no memory of what happened to them, and some have been sexually assaulted.

Using tranquilizers to deal with everyday difficulties causes the same problem associated with all depressant drugs: long-term dependence of a particularly stubborn kind. It is *very* difficult to wean people off benzodiazepines, since the withdrawal is unpleasant and dangerous. (Abrupt cessation can cause seizures and respiratory arrest.) Even though the health consequences of dependence on antianxiety drugs may be less severe than those of dependence on alcohol, the result is the same. There is no treatment of the underlying causes of anxiety, merely the creation of a legal drug habit.

The maker of Valium and Librium at one time pushed the idea

of using these drugs to treat alcoholics, and many doctors followed their advice. When the alcoholics drank less, the doctors imagined that they had achieved something, but all they had really done was to substitute one sedative-hypnotic for another. (One expert on alcoholism has called Valium "whiskey in a pill.")

Throughout history, doctors have relied on mood-altering drugs to deal with difficult patients. Psychoactive drugs change the way that people feel, satisfy patients' desire for medicine, and make doctors feel that they have been useful — or at least make the patients go away. A hundred years ago, opium and alcohol were the mainstays of medical treatment, along with cannabis (marijuana). At the turn of the twentieth century, doctors doled out cocaine for all sorts of complaints. Today, the benzodiazepines are some of the most widely consumed drugs. Certainly, they have their place in medicine, but prescribing them for weeks or months at a time to people who are anxious, depressed, or unable to sleep is symptomatic treatment of the worst sort.

Suggestions for Avoiding Trouble with Tranquilizers

1. Be aware that these drugs are strong depressants, similar in effect to alcohol, and can cause unpleasant reactions and dependence.
2. All of the cautions about downers apply to the minor tranquilizers as well.
3. If you take these drugs, whether by medical prescription or for fun, don't use them every day. Take them intermittently or occasionally to avoid falling into a pattern of habitual use.

GHB (Gammahydroxybutyrate)

GHB is an endogenous downer, made in small amounts in the brain as a metabolite of the sedative neurotransmitter GABA. In studies that go back to 1960, scientists have found it to be a safe inducer of sleep that does not cause tolerance or addiction. In the early 1990s, synthetic GHB became popular among body builders because it stimulates the pituitary gland to release growth hormone, which can help convert fat to muscle. The drug was unregulated, and manufacturers sold it through mail-order catalogs and to health food stores, where it was often described as a nutrient rather than a drug.

A teaspoon of GHB powder (about 2.5 grams), dissolved in warm water and taken on an empty stomach, produces within fifteen minutes a dramatic effect akin to alcohol or methaqualone intoxication. Most people find the effect pleasant, but in some individuals, especially with higher doses, GHB can cause nausea and marked incoordination, along with "hypersomnolence" (a kind of temporary stupor, in which people can stop breathing for periods). When GHB is combined with alcohol, adverse effects are more likely.

Unlike most psychoactive drugs and certainly most depressants, GHB increases rather than suppresses dreaming, and the sleep that it induces closely resembles natural sleep. It does not pose the risks of other drugs in this class, but users should be aware of the potential dangers of overdose, especially in situations that require full alertness, such as driving.

The Food and Drug Administration (FDA) has declared GHB to be a prescription drug and has halted distribution of it through the mail and through health food stores. The Drug Enforcement Administration has made it a controlled substance. In response, black-market manufacture of it has increased.

General Anesthetics

General anesthetics are powerful depressants used in surgery to make people insensible to pain. General anesthetics are gases or volatile liquids administered by inhalation through a mask placed over the face or tubes in the throat. Most are never seen outside operating rooms, but a few have been popular recreational drugs in the past, and one — nitrous oxide, or laughing gas — is still in common nonmedical use.

When inhaled, general anesthetics enter the blood very rapidly, depressing brain function within seconds. The stronger ones quickly produce complete unconsciousness, a state that lasts as long as the drug is administered and for a short time afterward. Like all depressants, general anesthetics can kill by shutting down the respiratory center and other vital functions. During surgery, therefore, a specially trained doctor or technician must monitor the administration of the drugs and the moment-to-moment condition of the patient.

In low doses, general anesthetics produce changes in consciousness similar to alcohol and sedative-hypnotics, and for many years people have experimented with general anesthetics to get high and to explore their minds.

Chloroform is one of the oldest drugs in this group. Since it is very toxic, it is no longer used. Years ago, people sometimes sniffed the fumes of liquid chloroform or swallowed small amounts in order to experience what disapproving critics called a "cheap drunk."

The era of surgical anesthesia began in 1846, when a dentist in Boston demonstrated that ether could safely render patients insensible to the pain of operations. Today, ether (or, more correctly, diethyl ether) is still widely used to induce unconsciousness before surgery. Ether is a volatile liquid, easily administered to people through breathing masks. It has a strong chemical smell, and its main disadvantage is that its fumes make an extremely explosive mixture with air. Great care must be taken when ether is in use to prevent violent explosions from accidental sparks or flames. Another disadvantage of ether is that overdoses of it rapidly put people into deep comas and stop their respiration.

Before 1846, surgery was horribly painful; patients had to be tied down, and their screams could be heard far from the operating room. The discovery of ether anesthesia revolutionized surgery. Even before this event — as long ago as 1800 — ether was a well-known curiosity; many people played with it just to experience its unusual effects on consciousness.

Ether parties were popular throughout the 1800s. People would gather for the express purpose of sniffing the fumes or drinking tiny doses of the liquid. When the drug was used in this way, its effects came on in a few minutes and ended within a half-hour. As might be expected, the reactions were highly variable, just as with alcohol. But although there are reports of a few "ether addicts" from this period, most people probably tried the drug only once or twice out of curiosity. A few writers of the time claimed that ether gave them profound insights into the nature of reality and even mystical revelations. (An 1874 book by the American physician Benjamin Paul Blood was titled *The Anesthetic Revelation and the Gist of Philosophy.*) Occasionally, people still experiment with ether, but if they like the effect that it gives, they tend to look for other drugs that are less toxic, don't smell as bad, and won't blow up so easily.

Nitrous oxide is such a drug. A gas with only a faint odor, it is relatively nontoxic and also nonflammable — although it will support combustion the way oxygen does and should be kept away from flames. Discovered in the late 1700s, nitrous oxide was quickly found to produce interesting changes in consciousness, as well as insensitivity to pain. Oddly enough, no one thought to use it in surgery until after the demonstration of ether anesthesia.

Nitrous oxide is a weaker drug than ether and the other general anesthetics; it does not produce complete loss of consciousness or anesthesia deep enough for major surgery. Nor is it so strong as to stop respiration. It is often used by itself in dentistry and minor surgery. In addition, many hospital anesthesiologists like to begin an operation by having the patient breathe nitrous oxide, then shift to ether and stronger drugs when the patient becomes totally relaxed and semiconscious.

People have been experimenting with nitrous oxide as a curiosity for the past two hundred years. Its effects, which come on within seconds, last as long as the gas is breathed, then disappear suddenly when it is stopped. Artists, writers, and philosophers have breathed nitrous oxide over and over in pursuit of elusive insights — revelations that seem overpowering under the influence of the gas but that evaporate as soon as normal consciousness returns. When the English poet laureate Robert Southey tried the gas at a nitrous oxide party in London in the 1790s, he commented afterward that the atmosphere of the highest of all possible heavens was no doubt composed of nitrous oxide.

On the other hand, many others have used nitrous oxide for less spiritual ends, especially to get hilariously intoxicated. The name "laughing gas" comes from a time when traveling medicine shows and carnivals would invite the public to pay a small price for a minute's worth of nitrous oxide. In these rowdy settings, the gas commonly produced silliness and uncontrollable laughter. Often, the laughers would stop in sudden confusion when the effect of the drug came to its abrupt end.

Today, nitrous oxide is available in many dentists' offices. Aware that people like to get high on it, some dentists give nitrous oxide even for routine procedures such as cleaning teeth. A fair number of tanks of the gas regularly disappear from hospitals and medical supply houses to find their way into the homes of recreational users. Many more people obtain smaller cylinders of the gas from restaurant suppliers, who use it to pressurize instant whipped cream cans. Some people even buy cans of instant whipped cream and attempt to get the gas out of the cans without the cream. Balloons of nitrous oxide are sold at some rock concerts.

Physicians and dentists have long considered nitrous oxide to be a safe pharmacological agent. Nevertheless, there is some evidence that excessive or prolonged use of it can damage the bone marrow and nervous system by interfering with the action of vitamin B-12. Moreover, its use in nonmedical settings presents several hazards that users should keep in mind. Breathing it directly from pressurized tanks is dangerous for two reasons. First, gas flowing from such tanks is very cold — cold enough to cause frostbite to noses, lips, and (most serious) vocal cords. Because users are anesthetized, they may be unaware of such injuries until it is too late. Second, because nitrous oxide does not support life, it should be mixed with oxygen if it is to be breathed for more than

a few minutes. People throwing private parties that feature nitrous oxide seldom supply oxygen tanks, and people have died of
asphyxiation by breathing straight nitrous oxide through a face
mask. One way to avoid these dangers is to fill balloons with nitrous oxide from a tank and inhale it from the balloons.

Further, nitrous oxide rapidly leads to complete loss of motor
control, and anyone who breathes it while standing will soon reel
about and fall down. Therefore, the only truly safe positions for
trying the gas are sitting and lying down. Serious injuries have resulted when people inhale laughing gas while standing in front of
an open window, driving a car, or operating machinery. Others
have been badly hurt by accidentally pulling a heavy tank of nitrous oxide over onto themselves while intoxicated.

People who breathe nitrous oxide for more than a few minutes
at a time may experience nausea, especially if they have just eaten.
They may also feel hung over for some time after. Addiction to nitrous oxide is a real possibility. Addicts may suffer serious mood
and personality changes in addition to the bone marrow and nervous system damage already mentioned.

Warnings About Nitrous Oxide

1. Never breathe nitrous oxide directly from a pressurized tank.
2. Never breathe nitrous oxide for more than a few minutes at a
   time.
3. Do not use nitrous oxide regularly over long periods of time.
4. Never breathe nitrous oxide while standing up or while doing
   anything that requires normal motor coordination.

Narcotics

The word *narcotic* comes from a Greek word meaning "stupor."
Stupor is a state of reduced sensibility that has given rise to our familiar adjective *stupid*. Narcotics are drugs that can produce stu-

pors by depressing brain function, but their depressant action is different from that of sedative-hypnotics or general anesthetics.

The parent of all narcotic drugs is opium, a dark gummy solid made from the opium poppy. Opium poppies are striking flowers, probably native to southern Europe and western Asia but now cultivated all over the world. As the flowers wither, the green pods, which contain many tiny seeds, begin to ripen and swell. If the pods are allowed to ripen fully, they turn brown and dry, whereupon the edible seeds can be gathered for use in cooking. While still unripe, the pods contain a milky juice that can be collected by letting it ooze from knife cuts. When dried, this juice is crude opium.

One of the oldest of all drugs, opium was used in prehistoric times; the ancient Greeks recognized its pain-relieving properties. Throughout history, opium has been an important item of commerce, and in some periods, it was the most widely used medical drug.

Opium can be taken by mouth or it can be smoked, but since smoking was unknown in Europe and Asia until Columbus brought news of it from the New World, opium smoking did not exist before 1492. Although the Chinese had used opium for centuries, widespread opium addiction did not occur in China until the early 1700s, when Portuguese sailors introduced the practice of mixing it with tobacco and smoking it. Many oral preparations of opium were made in the past. Two that survive into our own times are paregoric, a dilute tincture of opium combined with camphor, and deodorized tincture of opium, formerly known as laudanum, which is more concentrated.

Crude opium tastes very bitter and contains more than twenty different drugs, of which the most important is morphine. Named for Morpheus, the Greek god of dreams, morphine was isolated from opium in 1803 by a German pharmacist — an event that marked the beginning of the modern era of drug treatment, because it was the first time that an active principle was extracted from a drug plant. Morphine is prepared as a soluble white powder that can be mixed with water and injected into the body. Given by injection, it is a far more powerful and dangerous drug than when taken by mouth. Injection of drugs is relatively recent, dating only to the invention of the hypodermic syringe in 1853. Interestingly, the world's first morphine addict was the wife of the man who came up with that device.

Codeine (methylmorphine) is another natural constituent of opium. More active by mouth than other narcotics, it is a weaker pain reliever than morphine, and doctors frequently prescribe it today to treat moderate pain.

In the late 1800s, chemists began to experiment with variations on molecules of morphine and other compounds of opium. One of the drugs that they produced was heroin, a simple derivative of morphine first made available in 1898. Heroin (diacetylmorphine) is more potent than morphine — that is, it produces the same effect in smaller doses — but otherwise the two are very similar. In fact, the body promptly reconverts heroin to morphine. First marketed as a safe cough suppressant, heroin was declared to be nonaddictive, a claim that many users did not discover to be false until it was too late.

Drugs derived from morphine and other opium compounds are called opiates. Today, many hundreds of opiates are known; some are semisynthetic derivatives, like heroin, and others are purely synthetic, like Demerol. In general, all of the opiates produce similar effects. They differ from each other in potency, duration of action, how active they are by mouth, and how much mood change they cause relative to their physical effects. Opiates that are more potent, shorter acting, and more active by injection lend themselves more easily to abuse.

The main effects of opium and its derivatives are on the brain and the bowel. In the brain, these drugs cause relief of pain, suppression of the cough center, stimulation of the vomiting center, relaxation, and drowsiness. They may also cause mental clouding and inability to concentrate. Although they may induce sleep, they do not do so as reliably as the sedative-hypnotics. Some people become anxious, restless, and wakeful after taking opiates; others fall into a kind of twilight sleep marked by vivid dreams. Opium and opiates cause the pupils to contract, sometimes to tiny pinpoints; they also cause nausea and sweating, which can be profuse and uncomfortable. Larger doses often produce vomiting and depression of breathing. High doses of opiates, especially by injection, can cause death by stopping respiration, just like other strong depressants.

Because narcotics paralyze intestinal muscles, doctors prescribe them to treat diarrhea, particularly when it is accompanied by painful cramps. Regular use of opiates commonly results in chronic constipation.

In medicine today, narcotics are the main drugs used to treat severe pain. They are also prescribed to control bad coughs. In proper doses, when they are really needed, opiates are safe and extremely effective. Anyone who has experienced the rapid relief of terrible pain by narcotics knows what a blessing they can be. By allowing sick and injured people to take their mind off pain, to feel better, to relax and rest, narcotics can also indirectly promote healing. Opium and its derivatives have earned a secure place in treatment over many years of medical experience.

Yet narcotics have generated more fear and argument than any other class of drugs. The reason, of course, is their potential to cause addiction, a problem that was probably recognized even by ancient peoples when the only form available was crude opium, from poppies.

Narcotics addiction provides the classic model of drug dependence, and many of our current notions of drug abuse are based on it. For example, the fundamental principle that addiction consists of three features — craving for the drug, tolerance, and withdrawal — developed from observations of opiate addicts. Many popular beliefs about narcotics are untrue, however, and the whole subject is highly contaminated by prejudice and emotion.

There is no question that dependence on narcotics can develop quickly with repeated administration. When medical patients re-

> Laudanum gave me repose, not sleep; but you, I believe,
> know how divine that repose is, what a spot of enchant-
> ment, a green spot of fountains and flowers and trees in
> the very heart of a waste of sands!
>
> — Samuel Taylor Coleridge (1772–1834), from a 1798 letter
>   to George H. Coleridge

ceive morphine by injection every four hours, some degree of dependence can occur in as few as twenty-four hours. If the drug is
stopped even after a short period of use, mild withdrawal symptoms may occur — including sweating, nausea, weakness, headache, restlessness, and increased sensitivity to pain.

Tolerance for narcotics also develops rapidly and can reach
striking levels. The usual pain-relieving dose of tincture of opium
(laudanum) is twenty drops in a glass of water, repeated every four
to six hours if necessary. In England in the early 1800s, a number
of writers and artists were laudanum addicts with phenomenal
habits. The poet Samuel Taylor Coleridge, for example, consumed
as much as two *quarts* of laudanum a week. Thomas De Quincey,
best known for his *Confessions of an English Opium Eater,* took up
to eight thousand drops a day. Such doses would certainly kill people who have not built up their tolerance.

There is an important difference between tolerance for narcotics and tolerance for sedative-hypnotics. As we noted earlier, tolerance for the active dose of some sedative-hypnotics develops more
rapidly than does tolerance for the lethal dose, a process that can
— and does — result in fatal accidents. This is not the case with
narcotics, however, which makes them safer drugs. Heroin addicts occasionally die of overdoses, but such deaths result from
poor quality control in street supplies of the drug rather than from
the properties of heroin itself. (For example, an addict used to a
certain dose of impure street heroin may buy a packet of the drug

that, by accident, hasn't been cut as much as usual; injecting what he thinks is the right dose, he can unwittingly take too much.)

Withdrawal from narcotics is also less hazardous than withdrawal from sedative-hypnotics. Alcohol, downers, and the minor tranquilizers can produce violent withdrawal, marked by convulsions and, sometimes, death. Narcotic withdrawal can be intensely unpleasant, but it is not life threatening.

Also, the physical consequences of long-term narcotics use are minor compared with those of alcohol. People can take opium and opiates every day for years and remain in good health, provided they maintain good habits of hygiene and nutrition. There are many documented cases of opium and morphine addicts who, despite a heavy lifelong habit, survived to a ripe old age, remaining healthy to the end. Thomas De Quincey, for instance, who started taking laudanum for a toothache as a college student, died at seventy-four, still an addict. The worst medical effect of regular opiate use is severe and chronic constipation, which can be distressing but hardly compares to the cirrhosis of the liver and degeneration of the nervous system so commonly seen in chronic alcoholics.

Some addicts even claim that opiates help them to resist disease. Many heroin users say that they don't get colds or other respiratory infections as long as they take their drug. Since the symptoms of heroin withdrawal resemble those of a respiratory flu, it is possible that the drug somehow suppresses this kind of reaction. No one has investigated this claim of addicts; it would make an interesting subject of research.

The strong craving that characterizes opiate addiction has inspired many critics of narcotics to suggest that they destroy the will and moral sense, turning normal people into fiends and degenerates. Actually, cravings for opiates are no different from cravings for alcohol among alcoholics, and they are less strong than cravings for cigarettes, because nicotine is a more addictive drug.

The antisocial behavior of some opiate addicts seems more a function of personality, cultural background, expectation, and set-

> Junk is not a kick. It is a way of life.
>
> — **William S. Burroughs, from his novel** *Junky* **(1953)**

ting than of the drugs. Medical patients who become addicted to morphine in a hospital setting usually do not conform to stereotypes of addicts. They often have little difficulty separating themselves from narcotics once they are better and leave the hospital setting. People who can afford to support an opiate habit legally often lead normal lives while also being addicted. There are numerous cases on record of doctors and nurses who were opiate addicts yet seemed outwardly normal and fulfilled their professional and social responsibilities.

Apparently, a crucial difference exists between people who become addicted by chance or through medical circumstance and those who seek out opiates as a means of dealing with life's everyday difficulties. As with other depressants, serious dependence is most likely to develop when people use the drugs to screen out feelings of anxiety, depression, or boredom. Narcotics may be particularly seductive because they insulate people from discomfort and pain, seem to make time pass more rapidly, and create an inner world of security and comfort into which users can temporarily retreat from reality and its demands.

In the twenty-first century, heroin addiction is at epidemic levels worldwide. Thanks in no small part to America's "war on drugs," the world's supply of raw opium — already at record highs — is now expected to double every five years. The opium poppy grows well all over the world, but harvesting opium is very labor intensive. In countries with large pools of laborers willing to work for brief periods at low pay, no crop is more profitable than poppies. Converting raw gummy black opium into white powder heroin is also easier than you might think, much simpler than distilling alcohol, for example. It does not take much trouble or equipment to set up a heroin factory or to move it to another location if necessary. International heroin trafficking is a multibillion-dollar-a-year, mafia-controlled global system with supply routes connecting third-world producers with first-world consumers.

Heroin addiction condemns many people, especially the young, to unproductive lives of great hardship and cost to themselves and society and is rightly a cause for serious concern. It is not only the downtrodden poor of urban ghettos who become heroin addicts but the children of all social and economic classes and many of their parents as well. In opium-producing countries, populations of heroin addicts are steadily rising and contributing to the spread of serious communicable diseases like AIDS (acquired immune deficiency syndrome) and viral hepatitis.

When ordinary people look at heroin addicts, what they mostly see are victims of grinding social forces. Visible addicts tend to be in trouble, involved with crime, in poor health, purposeless, psychologically damaged, unhappy, and unable to get out of their grim predicament. Many of these conditions are more the result of society's blunders in trying to control the abuse of drugs than of heroin itself.

Heroin is often portrayed as the very worst of all possible drugs, a "devil drug," always productive of evil and somehow especially dangerous. In reality, it isn't very different from morphine, an accepted medical drug. Heroin is strictly illegal in the United States; even doctors cannot obtain it to use on patients. It is legal in England, however, where doctors do use it, sometimes with good results. Because it is more potent than morphine, it is sometimes a better pain reliever in small doses for people who are too sensitive to the nauseating effect of morphine.

By making heroin illegal, a society ensures that its heroin addicts will all be criminals. It is clear that drug laws have done nothing to discourage people from becoming addicts. There are more addicts than ever, and the kinds of addiction are worse than before those laws were passed.

The prohibition of opiates has spawned an ugly criminal underworld, given rise to powerful drug warlords, and led to the wide-

spread corruption of public officials. Campaigns to stamp out
heroin, while popular with politicians, have invariably had the opposite of their intended effect, ultimately causing more heroin to
enter the world market, not less. And because people are so susceptible to opiate addiction, when the supply of heroin increases,
so does demand for the drug.

Since the mid-1990s, opium production has reached unprece-
dented levels in southeast and southwest Asia, and opium farm-
ing has extended into new areas in central Asia and Latin America. This explosive growth has caused the street price of the drug
to plummet. In the mid-1990s, the street price for a gram of
highly adulterated material was about $1,000. Today users pay
$70 to $100 for a gram of heroin that may be 80 percent pure.

Because heroin is so abundant and cheap, new users tend to
snort or smoke the drug, rather than inject it into a muscle or vein,
which is more cost efficient. Heroin's reputation, long tainted
by its association with the hypodermic needle, is beginning to
change, especially among young people. They perceive heroin not
as a dangerous and unsavory "ghetto drug" but rather as a chic,
leading-edge intoxicant, and the taking of it has become something of a fashion statement. Although avoiding the needle, this
group is ingesting large quantities of high-purity heroin and pro-
gressing rapidly toward addiction.

The aspects of addiction that are attributable directly to heroin
have to do with the high potency of the drug, its short duration of
action, and the tendency for people to use it intravenously. (The
health problems associated with intravenous drug use are discussed in Chapter 12.) Heroin can be smoked (mixed with tobacco
or marijuana), snuffed up the nose, or injected under the skin,
into a muscle, or into a vein. By any of these routes, it is much
more powerful than by mouth. Oddly enough, most people who
try heroin for the first time, by whatever route, don't find it pleasant; more often than not, they experience little besides nausea,
sweating, and a general feeling of discomfort. After a few doses,
however — particularly when it is injected directly into the blood-

> There's nothing like a heroin rush. I started shooting her-
> oin when I was fourteen. It's just the most intense, wonder-
> ful feeling. I was always interested in getting high. One of
> my favorite ways when I was little was rolling down big
> hills. I did it over and over. Heroin has caused me a lot of
> problems. I'm scared of withdrawal, but I know I have
> to do it. I'm also interested in meditation and things like
> that, but I worry that I will always be tempted to feel the
> heroin rush again, because nothing else I've tried comes
> close to it.
>
> — seventeen-year-old woman, patient in a private addiction
>   treatment center

stream — some people experience an intense "rush" of good feeling that lasts for a few minutes, and then they become drowsy.

To hear heroin addicts talk about the intensity of this rush is
both fascinating and frightening. Some say that it is the most pleasurable sensation that they have ever felt, much more powerful
than orgasm. Users who get this experience from mainlining
heroin — not all do — find it hard to appreciate other kinds of
highs, especially nondrug highs, which tend to be more subtle.
The power of the heroin rush to make people uninterested in
other experiences and totally committed to heroin is so overwhelming as to be an argument against ever trying the drug at all.
One junkie expressed this sentiment in a much-quoted line: "It's
so good, don't even try it once."

Nonintravenous heroin doesn't give nearly as intense a rush
and so is less addicting. People who snort heroin can do so off and
on for long periods of time without becoming strongly addicted.
Even people who inject it subcutaneously ("skin-popping") can
sometimes avoid full-blown dependence, because they are able to
confine their use of the drug to occasional sprees. There is no
question that some users can mainline heroin only once in a

while, usually shooting the drug only in certain situations — to reduce anxiety in personal relationships, for example, or to feel good at weekend parties. In street jargon, this sort of occasional use of heroin is known as "chipping," and it seems that some lucky individuals remain successful chippers over months and even years. Unfortunately, a high percentage of chippers eventually go on to become addicted, so the practice is risky. Most junkies began as chippers, and many never thought that they would become addicts.

Once physical dependence develops, the need to avoid withdrawal becomes a powerful motive for taking more of the drug. Three to eight hours after her last dose, a heroin addict will begin to feel sick, and unless she takes another fix, these feelings will grow more and more intense.

Although heroin remains the most popular street opiate, many people have been discovering another poppy derivative — oxycodone. A semisynthetic opiate, oxycodone once was best known in combination forms: blended with aspirin as Percodan and with acetaminophen as Percocet, both widely prescribed drugs for pain. In 1995, the FDA approved Oxycontin, a more potent, time-release version of oxycodone. Aggressive marketing quickly made Oxycontin a blockbuster drug, and it soon became immensely popular with heroin addicts, who found that snorting the crushed pills delivered the full twelve-hour dose all at once. Since the late 1990s, Oxycontin has been rampant in areas where prescription drug abuse is common, such as working-class communities and Appalachia. In that region, it is known as "hillbilly heroin."

It is too bad that whole opium has disappeared from our society. When eaten, it is a much safer drug — less concentrated, longer acting, and easier to form a stable relationship with than other forms. Because it is a gummy solid, it cannot be injected directly into the bloodstream, and though people can certainly become addicted to it — as they did in England and America in the 1800s — the risk is much lower. Taking opium orally doesn't give a rush, and high doses cause unpleasant nausea, encouraging users to moderate their intake. Smoking opium puts drugs into the blood and brain more directly and has a higher potential for abuse.

Many junkies are as addicted to giving themselves intravenous injections as they are to the effects of heroin. Some addicts experiment with shooting other drugs, and some combine other drugs with their heroin. For instance, some addicts mix heroin and cocaine into a "speedball" that gives an intense euphoric effect. Of course, this practice is dangerous, much more so than combinations of stimulants and depressants taken by mouth.

Treatments of narcotics addiction are not very satisfactory. The physical component of an opiate habit can be broken fairly easily by withdrawing people gradually and treating symptoms as they develop. As with cigarette addiction, however, the relapse rate is very high, and junkies often go back to being junkies even after being drug-free for months or years.

Heroin maintenance — that is, supplying addicts with pure, legal heroin in some sort of supervised setting — has been proposed as a possible treatment, but our society, unwilling to abandon its prohibitionist mentality, has been unwilling to try it, even as an experiment. Instead, it has supported maintenance with methadone, a synthetic opiate that is active by mouth and has a long duration of effect. Oral methadone is an addicting narcotic but gives little euphoria. It does block the effect of heroin, however, and so may reduce a junkie's motivation to shoot heroin. Some addicts sign into methadone programs only to take a break from the street scene; after a time, they go right back to their old ways. Other addicts, if they are highly motivated, can use methadone programs to help them break their heroin habit once and for all.

The main advantage of methadone maintenance is that it is better than leading a criminal life. The real problem with it is that it doesn't go to the root of addiction. Nor does it show heroin users how to get high in more natural, less restricting ways. It offers

> The first opiate I ever took was codeine . . . It made me feel right for the first time in my life . . . I never felt right from as far back as I can remember, and I was always trying different ways to change how I felt. I used lots of drugs, but none of them really did it for me. Codeine was a revelation, and I've been an opiate user ever since . . . Opiates have caused me lots of trouble, but what they do for my head is worth it.
>
> **— thirty-four-year-old woman, rock singer**

them no help with the problems that led them to abuse heroin in the first place. All it does is substitute one narcotic for another; the addict remains an addict, albeit in a less destructive way.

(A new semisynthetic opiate called buprenorphine has recently gained attention as a treatment for heroin addiction. It blocks the high of heroin and can be given at higher doses than other opiates without suppressing breathing. The FDA approved buprenorphine in 2002. An advantage for addicts is that they can get this drug directly from doctors rather than only from special clinics.)

No matter how you look at it, heroin addiction limits your personal freedom. Like cigarette addicts, junkies cannot go anywhere or do anything without thinking about where their next fix is coming from. Unlike a cigarette addict, they cannot buy their drug for a reasonable price at the corner store, and they will become really sick if they cannot get it.

Nowadays, heroin use is becoming more and more common — invading affluent and respectable segments of society. In some circles, it is fashionable to try heroin or use it occasionally, particularly by means of "chasing the dragon," the practice of heating the drug on tinfoil and inhaling the vapors. Though the medical dangers of heroin have certainly been exaggerated, the risk of addiction is real.

If you do not try heroin, you will not use it. If you do not use it, you will never become addicted.

Many questions about opiate addiction remain unanswered. How much of it is biochemical and how much is psychological? Opiate molecules interact with special receptor sites on nerve cells in the brain. Might addiction be the result of suppression of the brain's own opiate-like molecules, the endorphins? Why do some people who try opiates find them so compelling that they go on to become addicts while others do not? Is this a matter of differences in brain chemistry or differences in personality? Unfortunately, the answers are still eluding scientists.

Given these uncertainties, it is impossible to say who is at greatest risk of addiction and who is not. There is no assurance that you will not become an addict once you start using opiates regularly, and there is no way to take the drugs *and* protect yourself from that possibility. Furthermore, once addiction develops, there is no reliable method of breaking it.

Precautions About Narcotics

1. Opium and its derivatives are powerful drugs that should be reserved for treating severe physical pain and discomfort.
2. Taking narcotics to reduce anxiety or depression, or just to feel good in the absence of physical pain, can easily lead to habitual use and addiction.
3. Never inject a narcotic into your body for nonmedical purposes.
4. If you ever try a narcotic intravenously and feel overwhelming pleasure, *never repeat it.*
5. If you begin to use narcotics regularly, by any method, and think that you can avoid going on to intravenous use and addiction, remember: most junkies thought that, too.

SUGGESTED READING

Drinking Occasions: Comparative Perspectives on Alcohol and Culture by Dwight B. Heath (Philadelphia: Brunner/Mazel, 2000) is an excellent look at different approaches to alcohol use around the world. Evelyn Waugh's *Brideshead Revisited* (Boston: Back Bay Books, 1999) describes the evolution of an English alcoholic. For a view of the use and abuse of alcohol on this side of the Atlantic, see *The Alcohol Republic: An American Tradition* by W. J. Rorabaugh (New York: Oxford University Press, 1979). Andrew Barr examines Americans' drinking habits in *Drink: A Social History of America* (New York: Carroll & Graf, 1999).

Several excellent films dramatize the problem of alcoholism. One classic is *The Lost Weekend*, about an alcoholic writer played by Ray Milland. *Days of Wine and Roses*, starring Jack Lemmon and Lee Remick, is an agonizing portrait of a pair of alcoholics whose lives are destroyed by drinking. An equally moving account of a person ravaged by alcohol (and other drugs) is *The Rose*, based on the life of the late rock singer Janis Joplin. *Only When I Laugh*, starring Marsha Mason as an alcoholic mother, takes a somewhat more humorous view of the problem drinker.

A novel in which downers figure prominently is Jacqueline Susann's *Valley of the Dolls* (New York: Bantam, 1967), which was also made into a movie. The minor tranquilizers and their manufacturers are strongly criticized in *The Tranquilizing of America: Pill Popping and the American Way of Life* by Richard Hughes and Robert Brewin (New York: Harcourt Brace Jovanovich, 1979, now out of print). One woman's personal story of addiction to Valium is told in *I'm Dancing as Fast as I Can* by Barbara Gordon (New York: Harper & Row, 1979).

A short but entertaining and informative book on nitrous oxide is *Laughing Gas (Nitrous Oxide)*, edited by Michael Sheldin and David Wallechinsky, with Saunie Salyer (revised edition; Berkeley, Calif.: And/Or Press, 1992).

The history of opium since ancient times is presented in *Flowers in the Blood: The Story of Opium* by Dean Latimer and Jeff Goldberg (New York: Franklin Watts, 1981). An excellent look at the history of opium in the United States is *Dark Paradise: A History of Opiate Addiction in America* by David T. Courtwright (Cambridge, Mass.: Harvard University Press, 2001). For a portrait of opium smoking in nineteenth-century China, see *The Fall of the God of Money* by Keith McMahon (Lanham, Md.: Rowman and Littlefield, 2002). Thomas De Quincey's

Confessions of an English Opium Eater, first published in 1821, is available in a modern edition (New York: Penguin, 1971). *The Opium Eater: A Life of Thomas De Quincey* by Grevel Lindop (Mineola, N.Y.: Dover, 1995) is a fascinating biography of the man who became world famous at the age of thirty-six, when his *Confessions* appeared. A number of novels concern opium, among them Charles Dickens's last work, *The Mystery of Edwin Drood,* written in 1870 and concluded by Leon Garfield (reissue edition; Oxford: Clarendon, 1987), and Wilkie Collins's classic from 1873, *The Moonstone* (reprint edition; New York: Dover, 2002). Louisa May Alcott wrote a short story about opium, "A Marble Woman: *or,* The Mysterious Model," collected in *Plots and Counterplots: More Unknown Thrillers of Louisa May Alcott,* edited by Madeleine Stem (New York: William Morrow, 1976). Barbara Hodgson's good book about laudanum is *The Arms of Morpheus: The Tragic History of Laudanum, Morphine, and Patent Medicines* (Buffalo, N.Y.: Firefly Books, 2001).

In *Heroin Century* (New York: Routledge, 2002), Tom Carnwath and Ian Smith elegantly present the sociological, medical, and historical facts about heroin. An excellent book on the history of that drug is *One Hundred Years of Heroin* by David F. Musto (Westport, Conn.: Auburn House, 2002). For treatment of heroin addiction, see the Drug Policy Alliance (www.drugpolicy.org/homepage.cfm) (last accessed April 2004) booklet *About Methadone* (New York: Drug Policy Alliance, 2003). The Drug Policy Alliance is the leading organization working to end the war on drugs. Another good book about treatment is *Methadone Maintenance Treatment and Other Opioid Replacement Therapies* by Jeff Ward, Richard P Mattick, and Wayne Hall (Amsterdam: Harwood Academic, 1998). A book that humanizes the perceptions of heroin addicts in modern times is *Tragic Magic: The Life and Crimes of a Heroin Addict* by Stuart L. Hills and Ron Santiago (Chicago: Nelson-Hall, 1992). Another interesting look at the drug is found in *The Politics of Heroin: CIA Complicity in the Global Drug Trade* by Alfred W. McCoy (Chicago: Lawrence Hill, 2003). Finally, see Edward J. Epstein's *Agency of Fear* (New York: Putnam, 1977), which details the dirty politics behind the Nixon administration's war on heroin and heroin addicts.

A number of creative writers have left us autobiographical records of their involvement with opium and opiates. One of the best is *Opium:*

The Illustrated Diary of His Cure by the French artist, writer, and filmmaker Jean Cocteau and translated by Margaret Crosland and Sinclair Road (Dufour Editions, 1990). Another is *Junky* by William S. Burroughs (New York: Penguin USA, 2003), which was first published in 1953 under the pseudonym William Lee. Ann Marlowe's memoir, *How to Stop Time: Heroin from A to Z* (New York: Basic Books, 1999), examines heroin addiction in the context of modern times. Aleister Crowley's *Diary of a Drug Fiend* (New York: Red Wheel/Weiser, June 1977) is an autobiographical novel about two English aristocrats addicted to heroin and cocaine. Alexander Trocchi's novel *Cain's Book* (reprint edition; New York: Grove Press, 1992) is a vivid picture of the often nightmarish world of the addict. *Heavier Than Heaven: A Biography of Kurt Cobain* by Charles Cross (New York: Hyperion, 2001) recounts the late rock star's struggles with heroin. One of the best-known novels about heroin addiction is Nelson Algren's *The Man with the Golden Arm* from 1949 (Seven Stories Press, 1999); it was made into a popular movie starring Frank Sinatra. Eugene O'Neill's play *Long Day's Journey into Night*, also made into a movie, is a harrowing account of his mother's addiction to morphine. Two recent films about the lives of heroin addicts are *Trainspotting*, based on the novel by Irvine Welsh, and *Permanent Midnight*, based on Jerry Stahl's memoir.

8. Psychedelics, or Hallucinogens

THE PLANTS AND CHEMICALS discussed in this chapter are some of the most colorful and controversial of all drugs. Some users have recommended them enthusiastically, claiming they are keys to understanding our minds and the origins of religious feelings. Many nonusers are fearful of them, regarding them as dangerous agents capable of driving people to insanity and suicide.

So heated is the debate over whether these drugs are good or evil that it's hard even to find a neutral name for them. When they first came to the attention of scientists in Europe and America in the 1950s, they were called *psychotomimetics,* based on the belief that they made people temporarily insane. (Psychiatrists now recognize that psychosis and the states induced by these drugs are very different.)

Many of the subjects who volunteered for the early research with these chemicals liked their effects very much. Unlike the doctors studying the drugs, the subjects thought of these drugs in positive ways and frequently wanted to repeat the experiences with friends outside the laboratory. As this group of devotees grew in number, they sought a more favorable name for the substances and came up with *psychedelics,* a word coined from Greek roots meaning "mind manifesting." The implication is that psychedelic drugs can develop the unused potential of the human mind.

At about the same time, the medical profession was using the term *hallucinogens* for the same compounds, meaning "causers of hallucinations." Since hallucinations are common symptoms of schizophrenia, this term carries the suggestion that the drug state is abnormal and unhealthy. The battle over names goes on. Recently, proponents have pushed for adoption of the term *entheogen*, meaning "creating God within." We will stick to *psychedelics* and *hallucinogens* and use the two interchangeably.

The substances in this class probably have the lowest potential for abuse of any psychoactive drugs. In purely medical terms, they may be the safest of all known drugs. Even in huge overdose, psychedelics do not kill, and some people take them frequently all their lives without suffering physical damage or dependence. In the right hands, they can bring about dramatic cures of both physical and mental illnesses. Yet these same drugs can cause the most frightening experiences imaginable, leaving long-lasting psychological scars.

Primitive people discovered hallucinogenic plants and began using them long before recorded history. Though many such plants exist, most are concentrated in North and South America, with heaviest use occurring among Indians of Mexico and Colombia. Very few natural psychedelics are native to the Old World, and there is little traditional use of them there. The main Old World psychedelic is a plant called iboga, whose root is made into a drink consumed in religious rituals by a few tribes of west Africa.

By contrast, hundreds of tribes of New World Indians use dozens of different hallucinogenic plants in tropical areas of North and South America. Among these people, the use of hallucinogens is tied to native practices of magic, medicine, and religion, particularly to the primitive religion called shamanism. In shamanism, specially trained individuals called shamans attempt to control the forces of good and evil within the tribal community by acting as a liaison for the human world and the spirit world. To contact the spirit world, shamans put themselves in an altered state of consciousness, often by consuming hallucinogenic plants. Shamans (or medicine men) also take psychedelics to see visions, and they use the visions to locate missing persons or lost objects and to diagnose illness. They often treat illness by administering psychedelics to sick people. In certain tribes, many people consume the plants at the same time in group vision-seeking rituals.

Most hallucinogenic plants taste bitter and cause nausea, vomiting, or other unpleasant physical symptoms at the onset of their effects. Then they induce unusual states of consciousness, altered perceptions, and fantastic visions that users see when their eyes are closed. However, visions and other sensory changes seem to come from taking these plants in particular ways and are by no means invariable occurrences. Indians who believe in the importance of visions and who eat hallucinogenic plants at night in front of a fire while chanting and praying under the direction of skilled shamans are much more likely to have visions than non-Indians who eat the same plants for purely recreational purposes. In fact, the mental effects of psychedelics are completely dependent on set and setting — on who takes them and why, where, and how.

Physical effects are more constant, because all of the hallucinogenic drugs have some common pharmacological actions. All of them are strong stimulants, for instance, causing increased brain activity and wakefulness. And they all stimulate the sympathetic nervous system, usually causing widely dilated eyes, a sensation of butterflies in the stomach, and feelings of cold in the extremities. The various psychedelics differ mainly in their duration of action and how fast their effects come on.

These substances fall into two broad chemical families. The first, called indoles, contain a molecular structure known as the indole ring and are related to hormones made in the brain by the pineal gland. The drugs in the second family lack the indole ring; instead, they closely resemble molecules of adrenaline and the amphetamines.

Indole Hallucinogens

LSD (Lysergic Acid Diethylamide, Acid, LSD-25)

LSD is the most famous of the psychedelics, probably the one that has been tried by the most people. It is a semisynthetic drug, not found in nature. A Swiss chemist, Albert Hofmann, first made it in a laboratory in 1938 from lysergic acid, a chemical in ergot, the fungus that attacks cereal grains, especially rye. At the time, he was interested in developing medical drugs from compounds in ergot. In 1943, Hofmann accidentally consumed some LSD and so discovered its psychoactivity. Beginning in the late 1940s, the Swiss pharmaceutical company he worked for supplied LSD as a research drug to doctors and hospitals throughout the world.

LSD is one of the most potent drugs known, producing its effects in doses as small as 25 micrograms. (A microgram is one millionth of a gram, and there are 28 grams in an ounce. An average postage stamp weighs about 60,000 micrograms.) An LSD trip lasts ten to twelve hours.

Throughout the 1950s, LSD remained mostly in the hands of researchers, especially psychiatrists. But many people who tried the drug found it so interesting that they publicized its effects and began taking it on their own. At first, most of the LSD in circulation was pure pharmaceutical material from the Swiss laboratory that originally made it. In the 1960s, when the psychedelic movement started in Europe and America, black-market LSD began to appear.

For the most part, people who took LSD in the early days had positive trips. They talked about experiencing powerful feelings of love, mystical oneness with all things, union with God, and a deeper understanding of themselves. Some described vivid sensory changes, such as seeing flowers breathe, objects shimmer with energy, and mosaic patterns appear on all surfaces. Such descriptions made other people, especially young people, eager to try the drug for themselves.

From the very first, however, it was apparent that not everyone who takes LSD has a good time. Some people had bad trips: they became anxious and panicky, afraid they were losing their minds and would be unable to return to ordinary reality. They almost always did return, when the drug wore off twelve hours later, but some of them remained depressed and anxious for days afterward, and a few had lasting psychological problems.

When people are panicked, they often behave in violent and irrational ways. In the 1960s, some bad trips on LSD may have led to accidents and suicides. Even though these cases were exceptional, the media seized on them and made it seem as if LSD were a new drug menace that threatened to turn teen-agers into lunatics.

Bad trips are more likely to occur when people take LSD in inappropriate settings, especially if they have never taken it before and if they take high doses. Throughout the 1960s, black-market LSD was unreliable, sometimes contaminated with other drugs, and since not many people were familiar with the effects of LSD, bad trips were common. By the 1970s, bad trips were rare, not because fewer people were taking the drug but because people had learned how to use it intelligently. They took reasonable doses in good settings (such as a familiar room or a peaceful field in the country), with friends who knew what to expect.

Street LSD comes in a bewildering array of forms, from small tablets of all colors and tiny transparent gelatin chips ("windowpane") to pieces of paper soaked in a solution of the drug or stamped with ink designs containing it. The windowpane and paper forms are likely to be the purest, since they are too small to contain contaminants.

Despite loud arguments and much bad publicity about the medical dangers of LSD in the 1970s, there is no evidence that it damages chromosomes, injures the brain, or causes any other physical harm. (Like other ergot derivatives, LSD causes contractions of the uterus. Pregnant women should not take it.)

Morning-Glory Seeds

The closest substance to LSD that occurs in nature is a chemical called ergine, or lysergic acid amide, found in the seeds of certain morning-glories. Indians in southern Mexico were eating morning-glory seeds for ritual purposes before the Spanish arrived, and some still use them today.

Not all the varieties of morning-glories available from seed companies are psychoactive. Of those that are, the best known are Heavenly Blue (with large blue flowers), Pearly Gates (white), Wedding Bells (pink), and Flying Saucers (blue with white stripes).

Because the concentration of LSD-like activity in the seeds of these plants is low, it takes a great many to produce a noticeable psychedelic effect, even up to several hundred, or a whole cupful. The seeds, which have hard, indigestible coats, must be cracked or ground up to release the drug. Also, they are mildly toxic, frequently causing nausea, vomiting, and other uncomfortable side effects. For these reasons, they are not popular; even the Mexican Indians who use morning-glory seeds regard them as a back-up psychedelic, taking them only when they can't get the hallucinogenic mushrooms that they prefer.

One species of morning-glory that is stronger than others is the Hawaiian Baby Woodrose, a creeping plant that covers many Hawaiian beaches and whose flowers are often dried and sold by florists. A dozen of the large, hard seeds will produce a strong intoxication, but they, too, frequently make people feel sick.

Devotees of psychedelics say that morning-glory seeds are definitely second rate, producing too much discomfort relative to the effects that they like. Another problem is that many commercial morning-glory seeds are now dipped in poisons to discourage people from eating them — sometimes without any caution to the buyer.

Mushrooms (Magic Mushrooms, Psilocybin)

Mushrooms are the most important natural psychedelics of southern Mexico, used in ceremonies so sacred that Indians carefully concealed them from Europeans until the twentieth century. It wasn't until the 1950s that descriptions of Mexican mushrooms came to the attention of the world. Soon after, botanists began to identify the mushrooms in use, and chemists found that their psychoactive properties came from psilocybin, an indole hallucinogen similar to LSD but with a shorter duration of action: four to six hours.

Mexican mushroom ceremonies are conducted by shamans,

usually women, and are held for purposes of treating illness, solving problems, foreseeing the future in visions, and putting people in contact with the supernatural world. They take place at night, by candlelight, and today are curious blends of shamanism and Roman Catholic ritual.

For some years, scientists believed that mushrooms containing psilocybin grew only in southern Mexico, and during the late 1960s and early 1970s thousands of people, mostly from Europe and North America, traveled there to take magic mushrooms in remote Indian villages. For a time, several Swiss pharmaceutical companies manufactured pure psilocybin, supplying it to researchers. As with LSD, some of this material eventually found its way to the street, but underground chemists never manufactured it because the synthesis is too costly.

As natural substances with a reputation for producing interesting experiences and fewer bad trips than LSD, magic mushrooms have been in great demand on the black market. For a long time, they were unavailable, though unscrupulous dealers often sold ordinary supermarket mushrooms laced with LSD and other drugs at high prices to unsuspecting customers.

Since the late 1970s, this situation has changed. In the first place, psilocybin mushrooms have been found in great numbers in many parts of the world. One of the principal species, called *Psilocybe cubensis,* is a large mushroom that grows in cow pastures in warm climates. It occurs in southeast Asia, in Central and South America, all along the Gulf Coast of the United States, and in many southeastern states. More than a dozen species of psychoactive mushrooms grow in the fields and woods of the Pacific Northwest. Some grow in Europe as well. In certain areas, the mushrooms are so abundant that collectors can easily gather enough for sale as well as for their own use.

Needless to say, collecting wild mushrooms of any sort requires knowledge and practice, because some mushrooms are very poisonous. No one should attempt to pick magic mushrooms without knowing how to recognize them.

Psilocybin mushrooms can also be cultivated. Although growing mushrooms from spores is much harder than growing green
plants from seeds, many people have mastered the technique.
Psilocybe cubensis is the easiest variety to grow; in recent years,
kits that include spores of the mushrooms have been widely sold
through the mail and in stores. Since the spores didn't contain
psilocybin, they weren't illegal. Taking advantage of this loophole
in the law, thousands of people have produced and distributed
magic mushrooms. Real, unadulterated mushrooms are now obtainable on the black market.

Both wild and cultivated mushrooms vary greatly in potency.
One medium-sized mushroom of a potent strain may give the
same effect as twenty of a mild strain. It is important, therefore, to
get advice on potency and dosage before eating mushrooms in order to avoid unpleasant effects from too-high doses.

Many wild mushrooms are hard to digest raw, and some are
mildly toxic until they are cooked. Psychedelic mushrooms may
taste better and are less likely to cause discomfort if they are dried
or lightly cooked before being eaten. Still, mushrooms are generally easier to take than the other hallucinogenic plants. One reason that people prefer mushrooms to other psychedelics is their
ease of consumption. Another is that the effects are shorter, usually ending after six hours, and therefore are less demanding on
the body. People usually feel sluggish the day after taking LSD or
other long-acting psychedelics. This is less common with mushrooms. (*Amanita muscaria,* the bright-red fly agaric [mushroom]
with white dots on the cap, is not a true hallucinogen. It is discussed in Chapter 10, along with other deliriant drugs.)

Ibogaine

Ibogaine is the active principle of the African hallucinogenic
plant iboga. Though the iboga root is almost unknown outside Africa, the pure drug can be made synthetically and sometimes appears on the black market. It is a long-acting psychedelic resembling LSD in effect, but it is an even stronger stimulant. Africans

who drink iboga in all-night ceremonies that include vigorous dancing may stay up the next day and night until the stimulation wears off. Eventually, they fall into a deep sleep.

Recently, ibogaine has been in the news as a potential new treatment for opiate addiction. After several heroin addicts discovered that a single ibogaine session eliminated their cravings for narcotics, scientists began to study this exotic drug in animals. Early reports suggest that it may work, but much more research is needed before ibogaine becomes an accepted treatment for addiction.

DMT (Dimethyltryptamine) and 5-MeO-DMT (5-Methoxydimethyltryptamine)

DMT is the drug responsible for the hallucinogenic properties of several plants used by South American Indians. It is a simple chemical closely resembling certain hormones made in the brain, and it is likely that the brain also produces DMT itself. DMT may be our own endogenous psychedelic. It is a compound easily made in laboratories; in the 1960s, synthetic DMT was sold in quantity on the black market.

DMT is peculiar among the psychedelics in that it cannot be taken by mouth; an enzyme in the stomach breaks it down before it can enter the bloodstream. Indians who use DMT-containing plants often prepare them as powdered snuffs. Users of the isolated, black-market chemical either smoke it or, less frequently, inject it intramuscularly.

A typical DMT snuff of South America is yopo, used by tribes of the Amazonian forests. It is made from the resin of a huge jungle tree, cooked down, dried, and pounded into a fine powder that the men blow forcefully into each other's noses through a long tube. Taken in this way, yopo causes a very intense intoxication within seconds but lasts only thirty minutes or less. While under its influence, Indians dance, sing, and see visions of gods and spirits.

Black-market DMT is usually a brown solid that smells like mothballs; users place tiny bits of it in the end of a joint made with marijuana, mint, or oregano in order to smoke the DMT. Sometimes a single inhalation of such a joint will be sufficient to initiate a five- to ten-minute trip of remarkable intensity. The effect may begin before the smoker can remove the joint from her or his lips and usually reaches its peak within the first minute. Some users, overwhelmed by visual hallucinations, lose all awareness of their surroundings. Fans of DMT say that it gives an ultimate psychedelic rush; needless to say, this experience can be quite frightening to someone unprepared for it.

After fifteen minutes, the strong effects subside, and after thirty minutes users again feel normal. Because of its short duration of action, DMT is known as the businessman's trip.

A close chemical relative of DMT is 5-MeO-DMT. It gives an equally powerful rush when smoked, but instead of visual hallucinations, the smoker experiences complete dissolution of reality. Some users describe this trip as "a rocket ship into the void." DMT and 5-MeO-DMT usually occur together in the plant sources of South American snuffs, but although synthetic 5-MeO-DMT has been readily available in North America, it has far fewer fans than its chemical cousin. The reason is that 5-MeO-DMT is often more frightening than delightful.

Nonetheless, a new natural source of this drug was discovered in the mid-1980s and has piqued the interest of many psychedelic explorers. The Sonoran Desert toad, a huge toad found in southern Arizona, produces large amounts of 5-MeO-DMT in its venom glands. These can be milked without harming the toad, and the venom can be dried and smoked. Users say the experience is gentler than smoking the synthetic drug.

Articles in tabloid newspapers have sensationalized this story, reporting inaccurately that people are licking toads to get high. Licking toads is dangerous. Only the Sonoran Desert toad's venom is psychoactive (other species are purely toxic), but it can cause serious poisoning if it gets in the eyes or mouth. Apparently, smoking destroys most of the toxic constituents while sparing the 5-MeO-DMT.

The dramatic effects of DMT and 5-MeO-DMT are good examples of the correlation between route of administration, duration of action, and intensity of effect. Short-acting drugs, introduced directly into the bloodstream by smoking or injection, tend to give rushes. Some people are especially fascinated by drug rushes, and, as we noted in the section on narcotics (pages 94–107), the pursuit of a rush can be the basis of addictive use.

That addiction to DMT and 5-MeO-DMT is unknown is due in part to the rapid development of tolerance for their interesting effects. When smoked regularly, they soon become ineffective. Another reason is the "high impact" of these experiences; they cannot easily be integrated into daily life in the way that highs of alcohol, marijuana, and cocaine can be.

All of the psychedelics share these characteristics. The body develops rapid tolerance for them, so that if you try to take them often, you do not get the results you want. Even people who really like these drugs don't take them every day, and most users save them for special occasions.

Ayahuasca (Yagé, Caapi)

Ayahuasca is a strong psychedelic drink made from a woody vine of the Amazon forests. Indians pound lengths of the vine with stones, then cook them in water for several hours, sometimes adding other plants to heighten the effect. They use the drink in all-night vision-seeking rituals with shamans or in large tribal ceremonies, such as coming-of-age rites for adolescent boys. The plant owes most of its activity to harmine, a drug rarely seen on the black market. Ayahuasca first causes intense vomiting and diarrhea and then a more relaxed and dreamy state than that produced by LSD; it lasts from six to ten hours. Indians say the spirit of the vine enters their bodies and makes them see visions of jungles and jungle animals, especially jaguars. Also, the drug is supposed to enable the Indians to see the future and communicate telepathically over great distances. Seeing visions while on ayahuasca, as with other psychedelics, depends very much on set and setting.

Curiously enough, the plant most commonly added to ayahuasca in making the drink is a leaf containing DMT. Indians say the addition makes for better and brighter visions. When scientists first learned of this practice, they dismissed it as useless on the ground that DMT is destroyed in the stomach. Further research has now shown that harmine inactivates the enzyme that destroys DMT. Combined with ayahuasca, therefore, DMT becomes orally active, and in this form it is a longer-acting, less intense drug that doesn't produce a rush.

How did Indians discover this remarkable combination of plants? Anthropologists and botanists say that the Indians did so by trial and error. Given the number of plants in the Amazonian jungles, that would mean a great deal of trial and error. The Indians themselves say they were inspired by visions — that the spirit of ayahuasca showed them the other leaves and the method of cooking the two together.

In recent years, religious groups using ayahuasca as a sacrament have proliferated in Brazil. Two of them — Santo Daimé and the União do Vegetal, or UDV — have attracted thousands of converts and remarkably little interference from Brazilian authorities. In both organizations, participants consume ayahuasca in groups, sing, dance, and commune with nature and the spirit world. Medical studies of members have found them to be physically and emotionally healthy. The UDV and Santa Daimé both report miraculous healings among participants. Missionaries from these organizations have brought the ceremonies and the psychedelic beverage to North America. At the same time, shamans, some imported from Peru and Colombia, others homegrown, have been conducting ayahuasca ceremonies for curious Americans, making this once unobtainable psychedelic plant quite easy to access. It has become extremely popular among intellectuals and seekers.

Hallucinogens Related to Adrenaline and Amphetamines

Indole hallucinogens make people feel high very rapidly. Typically, their effects begin in twenty to forty minutes and reach a

> My first vivid show of mescal colour effects came quickly. I saw the stars, and then, of a sudden, here and there delicate floating films of colour — usually delightful neutral purples and pinks. These came and went — now here, now there. Then an abrupt rush of countless points of white light swept across the field of view, as if the unseen millions of the Milky Way were to flow a sparkling river before the eye. In a minute this was over and the field was dark. Then I began to see zigzag lines of very bright colours.
>
> — from an essay by Dr. S. Weir Mitchell (1829–1914), an American physician and novelist who drank an extract of peyote in 1896

peak within the first hour or two. The drugs in this second family of psychedelics may also be felt quickly, but their onset is more gradual, reaching a peak after several hours. Some users find them less "electric" than LSD and its relatives, although in high doses the adrenaline relatives are more toxic than the indoles.

Peyote and Mescaline

Peyote is a small, spineless cactus with white, hairy tufts; it is native to the Rio Grande Valley in southern Texas and north-central Mexico. The tops of the cactus, cut off at ground level, dry into peyote "buttons" that retain their potency for a long time.

Some Indians in Mexico have used peyote since before recorded history, making long pilgrimages to the desert to collect it, then eating it in elaborate ceremonies. When the Spanish conquered Mexico, the Roman Catholic Church tried to stamp out peyote use, calling it sinful and diabolic, but to no avail. In the late 1800s, the use of peyote spread northward to Indians in the United States, who invented new rituals around it. As it moved north, peyote became even more popular; Indians of the midwestern plains organized a new religion based on it and helped spread its use all the way to Canada.

Not surprisingly, the explosion of this psychedelic movement among Indians generated intense opposition by non-Indians. Churches and government agencies charged that peyote made Indians crazy and violent; stories circulated of Indian men who, upon eating the cactus, axed helpless victims to death, while Indian women under its influence supposedly ripped off their clothes in a sexual frenzy. The similarity of the early peyote stories to those told about other psychoactive drugs is striking. (If there were high-rise tipis, newspapers would doubtless have reported peyote-crazed Indians jumping out of them, thinking they could fly.) The very same charges have been made about LSD, marijuana, heroin, cocaine, and PCP. Rarely have they had any basis in fact.

In response to official efforts to suppress the use of peyote, Indians organized formal churches and fought in court for their right to eat the cactus. The Native American Church began in this way. Eventually, it won its court battles and now boasts hundreds of thousands of members throughout North America. Indians have used peyote legally in Native American Church ceremonies, although most states have prohibited non-Indians from participating. However, this situation could change; a 1990 Supreme Court decision regarding the church declared that guarantees of religious freedom did not extend to the use of illegal drugs.

Native American Church "meetings" begin after dark, often in a tipi. The meetings take place around a fire, last all night, and include a great deal of singing, chanting, and praying, all coordinated by a leader, or "road man." Peyote is eaten throughout the night, and participants ask the spirit of the cactus to help make them better people, better able to deal with their problems. Sometimes the ritual includes elements of Christian worship. Church members tell many stories of illnesses cured as a result of peyote meetings, as well as cures of alcoholism, an addiction notoriously resistant to treatment by conventional means.

Peyote has a nauseating, bitter taste that is not soon forgotten. People who try it for the first time often find it hard to swallow, and it commonly causes vomiting. After an hour or two, the discomfort usually passes. Indians say that with repeated use, especially in religious ceremonies, nausea and vomiting do not occur. A typical dose of peyote is six to twelve buttons. Some users boil them in water to make a tea, and some non-Indians even take the tea as an enema in order to avoid the bad taste and effects on the stomach.

A persistent myth in the drug subculture is that the white hairs in the center of a peyote button contain strychnine, which is supposed to account for the sickness. In fact, there is no strychnine in peyote (or any other hallucinogenic plant), and the hairs are just cellulose, probably indigestible but certainly not poisonous. Peyote is bitter and causes nausea because it has a lot of drugs in it — more than forty separate compounds. Chief among these is mescaline, which accounts for much of the hallucinogenic effect.

Mescaline was isolated from peyote in the late 1890s. It is the only naturally occurring psychedelic in this family of adrenaline-related drugs. Throughout the twentieth century, a few artists, philosophers, and psychologists experimented with it on themselves, but there was no general demand for it until the psychedelic revolution of the 1960s. Then black-market mescaline began to appear. However, since the drug commands a higher price than LSD, many dealers sold LSD as mescaline. Real mescaline comes as long, needlelike white crystals; half a gram is the usual dose. The pure drug may cause initial nausea, though not as frequently as peyote. Its effects last up to twelve hours and generally resemble those of the whole cactus.

STP (DOM)

STP is a synthetic drug closely resembling mescaline in its chemical structure. It produces a twelve-hour intoxication with strong stimulation and may be less euphoric than mescaline. In the late 1960s, it was blamed for an epidemic of bad trips lasting many hours. The problem was overdose; some black-market tablets contained twenty times the recommended amount. This episode left STP with such a bad reputation that few people seek it out.

MDA (Methylenedioxyamphetamine)

Chemical variations of the amphetamine molecule have resulted in a number of synthetic psychedelics in this family. MDA is the oldest and best known, first made in Germany in 1910 but not discovered to be psychoactive until much later. In doses of 100 to 150 milligrams, it produces a feeling of physical and mental well-being. In the drug subculture, MDA is known as the "love drug" because it's supposed to inspire loving feelings in groups of people. Unlike mescaline, it rarely changes visual perceptions. Although it is a strong stimulant, chemically related to amphetamine, people who take it say that it calms them and promotes relaxation. Some users say it makes them more coordinated, more energetic, and better at physical activities. People often feel sluggish and drained of energy the day after taking MDA, and high doses can cause unpleasant muscular tension, especially in the face and jaw.

MDMA (Methylenedioxymethamphetamine, Ecstasy)

A newer drug, MDMA (usually called ecstasy, formerly known as XTC, MDM, and Adam), gives the same general effect as MDA but lasts four to six hours instead of ten to twelve. Because of its shorter duration of action, it is gentler on the body, with less day-after fatigue. Ecstasy has become one of the most popular recreational drugs in the world.

Taken by mouth in a reasonable dose (125 milligrams) and in a good setting, MDMA rarely causes bad trips. It has gained a strong reputation as an enhancer of empathy between people and an aid to psychotherapy and counseling. In other circles, it gained an equally strong reputation as a party or club drug, used especially in settings that featured "acid house" music and wild dancing. The acid house phenomenon grew quickly in Europe (particularly in the Netherlands and the United Kingdom) and in some American cities. It was then supplanted by the "rave," featuring synthesized music and light shows. Raves happened all over the world, from Israel to China, with millions of young people attending them and taking ecstasy as part of the experience. MDMA has also become very popular in the gay community and in gay bars.

For a number of years after its introduction, MDMA was an uncontrolled substance. It became illegal when government scientists charged that it caused permanent damage to certain nerve cells in the brain. Research has failed to support this idea, but the drug remains illegal, and strange stories circulate about it. One is that it causes the spinal cord to liquefy.

There is no truth to these stories, but both MDA and MDMA can cause bad reactions at high doses. Some people snort them or (rarely) inject them intravenously, intensifying their action and potential for harm. Combining these drugs with alcohol or other depressants also increases the possibility of adverse effects. As sexual drugs, both compounds enhance the pleasure of touching, but they interfere with erection in men and with orgasm in both men and women. A few cases of dependence on MDMA have been reported; they resemble cases of amphetamine dependence.

Some users risk hyperthermia (overheating) from taking MDMA in hot, poorly ventilated clubs, engaging in intense dancing, and not drinking enough water. The drug does not cause hyperthermia; overexertion and dehydration in hot rooms do.

There is some evidence that the popularity of MDMA has begun to wane. Its enthusiasts say that no other drug gives quite the same experience, and some physicians and psychotherapists are still trying to convince the government that it should be made available for both research and treatment. The most common complaint about it from long-time users is that sensitivity to day-after fatigue seems to increase as people get older. Some people say they have sworn off the drug entirely because they feel so run-down after using it and find themselves more susceptible to colds, herpes outbreaks, and infections.

Designer Psychedelics

A number of other synthetic drugs exist in this series, with names like MMDA, TMA, PMA, 2CB, 2CT2, 2CT7, and so forth. Since they are custom-made by psychedelic chemists, writers often refer to them as "designer psychedelics." Most are pharmacological curiosities, rarely seen on the street. They differ from other drugs in this section and from each other in duration of action, euphoric potential, and tendency to affect visual perception.

2CB was first made in 1974 and is one of the more popular designer psychedelics. A close relative of mescaline, it produces a six-hour high that users say feels like a middle ground meeting of that drug and MDMA. That is, it gives the relaxed, centered, empathetic effect of ecstasy with more of the visceral stimulation and visual changes of mescaline. 2CB is quite potent; a typical dose is only 15 to 20 milligrams (an amount of white powder about the size of a match head). Some users snort the powder to get immediate effects. It is easy to take too much, and overdoses are unpleasant, commonly marked by nausea and incoordination. Unlike MDMA, 2CB causes minimal day-after fatigue.

A Psychedelic in a Class by Itself

Salvia divinorum is a Mexican sage with a long history of use by native peoples in the same region where magic mushrooms are used traditionally. In the past few years, it has become surprisingly popular in the United States, with living plants, dried leaves, and extracts all easy to obtain. The active principle is a substance called salvinorin-A; it is a potent inducer of visions but is unrelated to any of the other hallucinogenic drugs discussed in this chapter.

As a purified compound, salvinorin-A is active in microgram amounts, which makes it almost as potent as LSD. It can be vaporized and inhaled, but the effects can be overpowering and quite unpleasant if taken in this manner. It is much better taken by mouth or under the tongue. Better still is to smoke the leaves or soak them in water to make a tea. When smoked, *Salvia divinorum* produces effects that come on quickly, peak for five to twenty minutes, then subside. Oral preparations take effect more slowly and last longer, up to three hours.

Experiences vary from subtle alterations of consciousness to full-blown psychedelic trips. At moderate to high doses, users report profound peace, feelings of connection with the universe, vivid imagery, dramatic time distortion, encounters with beings, and travel to other places, times, and dimensions.

Scientists have no clue how *Salvia divinorum* and salvinorin-A work in the brain. The substances appear to be safe, but we have no data on long-term or repeated use. At this writing, only Denmark and Australia have laws against this exotic psychedelic.

Benefits and Risks of Psychedelic Drugs

Bad trips are the greatest danger of hallucinogenic drugs. Most bad trips are related to set and setting, but they also depend on dose and quality of the drug. Since legal sources of pure psychedelics do not exist, users are faced with the problem of not knowing what they are buying. All powders, pills, and capsules are suspect; only mushrooms and peyote buttons are likely to be genuine. Even good psychedelics can cause unpleasant effects if you take too much of them, and with street drugs it's not easy to determine how much is enough.

Psychedelics do not necessarily produce any particular mood or state of mind. They act as intensifiers of experience. If you take them when you are elated, they may make you super-elated. If you take them when you are depressed, they may make you super-depressed. If you take them with a friend you feel totally comfortable with, they may deepen your friendship. If you take them with someone you feel uncomfortable with, they may intensify that discomfort to an unbearable degree. Therefore, if you are going

> You get out of the drug experience only what you put into
> it. The "Otherworld" from which you seek illumination is,
> after all, only your own psyche.
>
> — Peter Furst, anthropologist, from his book *Flesh of the Gods* (1972)

to take these drugs, you must be extremely careful about when,
where, and with whom you take them.

Because hallucinogens are strong stimulants that make people
feel very different from normal, they cannot easily be combined
with everyday activities. They demand that you set time aside from
your routine. Their abuse potential may be low precisely because
they make this demand. Other stimulants allow people to perform
ordinary activities, but it is not appropriate to take psychedelics
and expect to go about your business.

Some people who take psychedelics, especially LSD, later become worried about flashbacks — brief recurrences of psychedelic symptoms that may include visual changes and "spacy" feelings. Anxiety about these experiences is more the problem than
the flashbacks themselves. Actually, many people who have never
taken hallucinogenic drugs also have flashbacks or experiences
very much like them, which may mean that these are normal
events in the nervous system. The best treatment for flashbacks is
reassuring the tripper that nothing is seriously wrong. As people
worry less about their symptoms, they pay less attention to them,
and soon the flashbacks themselves fade away.

The benefits that people have claimed from using psychedelics
range from cures of mental and physical problems to increased
appreciation of the beauty of nature to better understanding of
themselves to just having a good time. Some medical doctors
and psychologists have been able to cure patients of serious emotional disorders by means of psychedelic therapy. There is an ex-

tensive literature on the value of using these substances occasionally and intelligently (see the Suggested Reading at the end of this chapter).

Suggestions and Precautions for the Use of Hallucinogenic Drugs

1. Know your sources. Many fake and adulterated versions of psychedelics are sold on the street.
2. Do not attempt to pick wild psilocybin mushrooms without knowing what you are doing.
3. Cultivated psilocybin mushrooms vary greatly in potency. Get advice about dose before eating any.
4. Do not take psychedelics unless you are in good physical and psychological shape.
5. If you are trying one of the hallucinogenic drugs for the first time, take it with an experienced companion.
6. Take psychedelics only in a comfortable setting when you have no responsibilities for at least the next twelve hours.
7. Remember that you may feel tired and drained of energy the following day.
8. Do not take psychedelics on a full stomach; you are less likely to feel nausea or other discomfort if your stomach is relatively empty.
9. Do not combine psychedelics with other drugs. However, the interesting effects of psychedelics sometimes wear off while their stimulation continues. If you feel agitated, restless, and unable to sleep at the end of an experience with one of these drugs, it may be appropriate to take a hypnotic dose of a sleeping pill or minor tranquilizer.
10. Remember that hallucinogenic drugs can affect perception and thinking. Do not drive, operate machinery, or engage in hazardous activities while under their influence.
11. Take psychedelics by mouth. They are more likely to cause bad reactions by other routes of administration.

12. If you take MDMA in a club setting, be sure to drink plenty of water and get enough fresh air.

13. The best experiences with these drugs result from saving them for special occasions and the right circumstances. Taking psychedelics just because they are available is less likely to produce valuable results. Taking them to get yourself out of a bad mood may intensify that mood. Taking them frequently and carelessly reduces their potential to show you interesting aspects of yourself and the world around you.

SUGGESTED READING

Probably because they are so colorful and controversial, psychedelics are the subject of more books than most of the other categories of drugs. Many of the books are good.

In collaboration with Albert Hofmann, the discoverer of LSD, Richard Evans Schultes has written *Plants of the Gods: Origins of Hallucinogenic Use* (reprint edition; Rochester, Vt.: Inner Traditions International, 1992), a large and beautifully illustrated work on the world's psychedelic plants. Peter Stafford's *Psychedelics Encyclopedia* (third edition; Berkeley, Calif.: Ronin, 1992) covers the chemical psychedelics as well as plants and is filled with historical information, descriptions, pictures, and anecdotes. *PIHKAL: A Chemical Love Story* by Alexander Shulgin, Ann Shulgin, and David Nichols (Berkeley, Calif.: Transform Press, 1991) is an unusual autobiographical account by a renowned psychedelic chemist that includes detailed descriptions of many designer psychedelics related to mescaline and MDMA. *TIHKAL: The Continuation* is another book on psychedelics by Alexander and Ann Shulgin (Berkeley, Calif.: Transform Press, 1997).

A more comprehensive and scholarly work is *Psychedelic Drugs Reconsidered* by Lester Grinspoon and James B. Bakalar (third edition; New York: Bookworld Services, 1997); it contains a complete bibliography and discusses the uses of hallucinogens in psychotherapy.

Albert Hofmann, together with R. Gordon Wasson and Carl A. P. Ruck, wrote *The Road to Eleusis: Unveiling the Secret of the Mysteries* (reprint; New York: William Dailey Antiquarian, 1999), a fascinating speculation on the use of a psychedelic potion in ancient Greek religious rites. *Storming Heaven: LSD and the American Dream* by Jay Stevens (New York: Grove Press, 1998) is a fascinating account of the place of LSD in American culture. A good book on how LSD can influence creativity and imagination is *LSD, Spirituality, and the Creative Process* by Marlene Dobkin De Rios et al. (Rochester, Vt.: Park Street Press, 2003). See also *The Politics of Ecstasy* by Timothy Leary (Berkeley, Calif.: Ronin, 1990).

An excellent book on magic mushrooms is Paul Stamets's *Psilocybin Mushrooms of the World: An Identification Guide* (Berkeley, Calif.: Ten Speed Press, 1996); many of Stamets's other excellent books about mushrooms are available from www.fungi.com (last accessed April 2004). Terence McKenna's *Food of the Gods* (New York: Bantam, 1992) is an entertaining and articulate speculation on the influence of psilocybin on human evolution and the value of the psychedelic experience.

The best descriptions of the effects of ayahuasca appear in F. Bruce Lamb's *Wizard of the Upper Amazon: The Story of Manuel Córdova-Rios* (third edition; Berkeley, Calif.: North Atlantic Books, 1986). Other good books on the subject are *The Ayahuasca Reader: Encounters with the Amazon's Sacred Vine,* edited by Luis Eduardo Luna and Steven F. White (Santa Fe, N.Mex.: Synergetic Press, 2000), and *Ayahuasca: Human Consciousness and the Spirits of Nature* (New York: Thunder's Mouth Press, 1999), edited by Ralph Metzner et al.

Shabono by Florinda Donner (San Francisco: Harper, 1992) is the gripping story of a young American anthropologist who lived with a South American Indian tribe; the Indians value altered states of consciousness and use a DMT snuff. See also *DMT: The Spirit Molecule: A Doctor's Revolutionary Research into the Biology of Near Death and Mystical Experiences* by Rick Strassman, M.D. (Rochester, Vt.: Inner Traditions International, 2001).

The best recent work on peyote is Edward F. Anderson's *Peyote: The Divine Cactus* (second edition; Tucson: University of Arizona Press, 1996). For an analysis of the role of peyote in American Indian cultures by a historian who has studied the subject for fifty years, see Omer C. Stewart's *Peyote Religion: A History* (reprint; Norman: University of Oklahoma Press, 1993). Aldous Huxley provided many excellent writings on mescaline and other psychedelics. His most famous work on the subject is his 1954 essay *The Doors of Perception* (New York: Harper & Row, 1970).

Of the many recent writings on MDMA (ecstasy), the most important and complete book is *Ecstasy: The Complete Guide: A Comprehensive Look at the Risks and Benefits of MDMA* by Julie Holland, M.D. (Rochester, Vt.: Park Street Press, 2001).

For information on *Salvia divinorum,* see *Salvinorin: The Psychedelic Essence of Salvia Divinorum* by D. M. Turner (Tennessee: Panther Press, 1996).

Research information on psychedelics is available from MAPS, the Multidisciplinary Association for Psychedelic Studies, at www.maps .org (last accessed February 2004).

So far, the only movie to focus on the psychedelic experience in a positive way is *The Emerald Forest.* A more distorted picture is presented in *Altered States. Easy Rider* and *Midnight Cowboy* both have brief hallucinatory scenes. A visually interesting film about psychedelics is Terry Gilliam's *Fear and Loathing in Las Vegas,* based on the book of the same name by Hunter S. Thompson.

9. Marijuana

MARIJUANA is an ancient drug, used since prehistoric times in parts of the Old World. It is a product of the hemp plant, *Cannabis sativa*, a species that also provides a useful fiber, an edible seed, an oil, and a medicine. That is a lot for one plant to do, which explains why it has always been an important cultivated crop. Cannabis is probably native to central Asia. It tends to grow in waste places — along roadsides, in abandoned lots — around camps and settlements and has been associated with human beings for so long that it is unknown in a truly wild state.

The intoxicating properties of hemp reside in an aromatic, sticky resin exuded by the flowering tops, especially the tops of female plants. The strength of a preparation of hemp depends on the resin content; some strains produce a great deal of resin, others little. If whole plants are chopped up, leaves, stalks, and all, the resin-rich tops will be diluted by much inert material. Carefully cultivated female tops, gathered before the seeds form, are sticky to the touch with resin, highly aromatic, and very potent. The resin itself can be collected and pressed into cakes or lumps; that is hashish. Also, the resin can be extracted with solvents and concentrated into a thick, oily liquid called hash oil. Any of these preparations can be either smoked or eaten.

Marijuana is unique among the psychoactive drugs, in a class by itself. The chemicals it contains resemble no other drug molecules. Unlike most of the substances discussed in this book, marijuana molecules are insoluble in water but very soluble in oil. Therefore, they are absorbed unevenly when eaten, and they stay in the body for a long time because they accumulate in body fat. Marijuana is neither a stimulant nor a depressant but has some features of both. Many people regard it as a mild psychedelic, but its effects are different from those of the true hallucinogens, and it is not necessarily mild. Moreover, the abuse potential of marijuana is considerably higher than that of psychedelics, because it can be used frequently or continually in combination with everyday activities.

As a psychoactive drug, cannabis has a much longer history in other parts of the world than it does in Western countries. Europeans and Americans grew the plant exclusively for its fiber for many years, and even when tincture of cannabis was widely used in Western medicine in the 1800s, few people took it to get high or reported that they felt high when they did take it. The knowledge of how to smoke hemp was probably brought to Brazil by black slaves who used the plant in Africa; the practice traveled north to Mexico and, finally, reached the United States.

Marijuana smoking began in the United States after World War I. Introduced by Mexican migrant workers, it caught on first among black people in southern cities. Many of its early users were musicians. Over the years, it spread to other subgroups but was not associated with the white middle class until the 1960s, when it became a prominent symbol of the youth movement on college campuses. Since then, it has grown steadily more popular and today is the most widely used of all the illegal drugs. From the very first, marijuana — which is known by many slang names, including pot, grass, weed, and dope — provoked a great deal of contention, mostly as a result of its associations. It was the drug of minority races and deviant subcultures even before it got mixed up with hippies and revolutionaries. Despite its status as the most widely used illegal drug today, the dominant culture still views it as a dangerous drug, worse than alcohol and tobacco, likely to lead to heroin.

In this highly charged atmosphere, arguments about marijuana tend to be more political than factual. And because pharmacologists and medical doctors are just as caught up in the politics of marijuana as other people, it's difficult to get neutral information about the drug. Much marijuana research sets out to prove pre-conceived ideas, and much of it is not worth reading.

Politics aside, the effects of marijuana are hard to describe, be-cause they are so variable — more so than those of other drugs. Some of this variation has to do with set and setting, but some is inherent in the drug.

People who smoke marijuana for the first time often feel noth-ing at all, even if they take high doses of strong pot. As with other psychoactive substances, people have to learn to associate changes of consciousness with the physical effects of the drug. Compared with other drugs, however, the physical effects of marijuana are not spectacular. It makes the heart beat somewhat faster, causes the mouth and eyes to become dry, and reddens the whites of the eyes. Of these, the most noticeable change is the dryness of the mouth. Only people who wear contact lenses are likely to notice the dryness of the eyes. Increased heart rate is easily ignored, al-though it can become the basis of a panic reaction in anxious first-time users, who may interpret it to mean that they are having a heart attack.

When people learn to get high on marijuana, their early experi-ences with it are often quite lively. Everything may strike them as funny, and all sensory experiences become novel and interesting. Listening to music, eating, and making love can become more than usually absorbing. Time seems long and drawn out. People sometimes have strange illusions, such as seeing a room expand or feeling as though their legs have become enormously long.

With repeated use, these remarkable effects tend to fade away. Regular users may find that pot makes them relaxed or more so-ciable without greatly affecting their perceptions or moods. Very heavy users usually feel little from the drug, often smoking it sim-ply out of habit.

Bad reactions to marijuana are more likely when high doses of strong material are taken in bad settings, especially by inexperienced users. Most are simple panic reactions, easily treated with reassurance that everything will be all right as soon as the drug wears off. The effects of smoking marijuana usually diminish after an hour and disappear after two or three hours. Some people, if they have smoked a lot of pot, feel tired or "fuzzy" the next morning.

Some users find that marijuana stimulates them and keeps them awake at night; others use it to help them fall asleep. It makes some people depressed and irritable, and others groggy for several hours. Some kinds of pot may be more sedative than others. In recent years, stronger and stronger marijuana has become available, as breeders have selected strains for greater potency. Some of the most potent strains (like the "skunk weeds" from northern California and British Columbia) are as strong as hashish and can be disorienting to people who are not used to them.

Taken by mouth, rather than smoked, marijuana is a more powerful drug, slower to come on, with longer-lasting effects. Because the resin is insoluble in water, marijuana tea is not very effective. But the crude drug can be added to food, and the active principles are easily extracted in alcohol or fat. Although some users like to eat cannabis, most prefer to smoke it because it's less trouble, and the effect comes on very fast. The main problem with oral use is the risk of overdose. Since the stomach absorbs the drug unevenly, the right dosage is hard to estimate, and it's easy to take too much. Overdoses of cannabis are unpleasant, though not dangerous medically. They can make people extremely disoriented and delirious, as if suffering from a high fever, and are often followed by stupor and hangover. Perhaps because oral use requires more preparation and produces stronger effects, people who eat marijuana are less likely to become dependent on it than people who smoke it.

Whether they eat it or smoke it, users frequently combine marijuana with other drugs, such as alcohol, downers, stimulants, and even psychedelics. The effects of these combinations are not predictable, depending more on the individual than on the drugs. Because marijuana is not as powerful or as toxic as most of the other drugs, there is no special pharmacological danger in mixing it (as there is, say, in mixing alcohol with downers). Still, users should be aware that combinations that they are not used to may disagree with them and may produce unexpectedly strong effects.

The medical safety of marijuana is great. It does not kill people in overdose or produce other symptoms of obvious toxicity. Occasional use is no more of a health problem than the occasional use of alcohol.

Smoking marijuana regularly can, over time, significantly irritate the respiratory tract, causing chronic, dry coughs that resemble the coughs of some cigarette smokers. Further, marijuana smoke may contain more tars than tobacco smoke and can probably produce lung and bronchial disease in susceptible individuals. The risk depends on how much users smoke over how long a time. A few users avoid the irritation from smoke by consuming marijuana from a vaporizer, a device that heats the plant material but only to temperatures well below the point of combustion.

Aside from respiratory irritation, heavy marijuana use does not seem to cause other medical problems. Of course, warnings of the medical dangers of cannabis have been well publicized, with reports of everything from brain damage to injury to the immune and reproductive systems, but these are based on poor research, often conducted by passionate foes of the drug. Studies of populations that have smoked cannabis for many years do not reveal obvious illnesses that can be linked to marijuana.

Much has been made of the fact that tetrahydrocannabinol, or THC, the most active chemical in cannabis resin, accumulates in body fat, staying around for weeks after the last dose of marijuana is smoked. Although this is true, and it is very different from the pattern of quick elimination of water-soluble drugs, it is not a problem in itself. If THC were a very toxic drug, its persistence in body fat would be cause for concern, but THC and marijuana are less toxic than most of the drugs discussed in this book.

(Marijuana may be quite toxic if it is contaminated with para-

> I started dealing dope 'cause it was the only way I could afford to buy dope. Now I do it for the money.
>
> — sixteen-year-old man

quat, a very poisonous chemical herbicide used to kill unwanted plants. In 1975, American drug enforcement authorities began encouraging officials in Mexico to spray this poison from helicopters on the illegal marijuana fields of that country. The growers soon learned that if they harvested their pot immediately after it was sprayed, it would still look healthy and could be sold to dealers as usual. In this way, paraquat-contaminated Mexican marijuana began to find its way to users in the United States. The exact dangers of smoking paraquat are unclear, but it is certain that it cannot be good for you; the only question is how bad it is. Apparently, it can cause serious lung damage over time and may affect other organs as well. There is no easy way to spot paraquat on a sample of pot, but some drug testing labs can analyze for it. Although public outcry put an end to American support for the Mexican program, the drug enforcement authorities have continued to try to use paraquat on marijuana fields in other countries.)

Psychological problems related to regular use of marijuana are also controversial. Opponents of the drug charge that it interferes with memory and intellectual functioning and leads to an amotivational syndrome in which people lose their initiative and will to work. There is no question that young people who lack motivation often smoke a lot of pot and do very little else, but it is doubtful that marijuana made them that way. Heavy pot smoking is more likely to be a symptom of amotivation than a cause, and those same young people would probably be wasting their time in other ways or with other drugs if pot were not available.

As for its effects on memory and intellect, regular users often say that marijuana makes their minds fuzzy and can interfere

> If you can remember the sixties, you weren't there.
>
> — Robin Williams, actor

with memory. These effects disappear when people cut down on their use of the drug or stop using it altogether.

Dependence on marijuana certainly occurs and has become more common as use of the drug has increased. It does not exactly resemble dependence on any other psychoactive drug. At its worst, marijuana dependence consists of chain smoking, from the moment of getting up in the morning to the time of falling asleep — a pattern similar to that of many cigarette smokers. But dramatic withdrawal syndromes don't occur when people suddenly stop using marijuana, and craving for the drug is not nearly as intense as for tobacco, alcohol, or narcotics.

Tolerance for marijuana also occurs. Even the strongest varieties seem to lose their power if people smoke them day in and day out. This leads heavy users to keep searching for more potent pot so that they can feel stoned again. In fact, all they really need to do is cut back on their frequency of use; even a twenty-four-hour break from the routine of smoking all day long will allow a heavy user to become sensitive again to the psychoactive properties of marijuana.

Although dependence on marijuana has fewer physical components than dependence on more toxic drugs, it can still be very hard to break and very upsetting to people who find themselves caught up in it. Some heavy users are unable to stop smoking, even though they no longer get useful effects from pot and, in fact, get effects that they actively dislike, such as strong sedation and chronic coughs. There are now self-help groups modeled on Alcoholics Anonymous for people with unwanted marijuana habits.

Marijuana dependence can be sneaky in its development. It

Eventually, I became a daily pot smoker, sometimes starting in the morning. It was my main way of relating to other people. However, I started getting less and less effect from it that I liked. In fact, it began to make me groggy and sleepy most of the time and also gave me a cough. These unwelcome effects got worse and worse until I realized I would have to stop using pot. So I made a resolution to quit completely.

Well, it surprised me to find that wasn't so easy. It took me three years of trying before I really gave up smoking marijuana, even though I no longer got pleasant effects from it. I never realized how much of a habit I had and how hooked I was on it.

— forty-one-year-old man, lawyer

doesn't appear overnight like cigarette addiction, or in a matter of weeks like heroin addiction, but rather builds up over a long time. In most cases, people begin smoking pot only in special, usually social, situations. At first, because the drug causes such strong effects, they cannot imagine smoking it at other times. With increasing use, however, tolerance develops, and also people learn to adapt to being high. Soon they can perform normal activities while under the influence of marijuana. Users may then begin to smoke during the day, perhaps by themselves. With time, and unless precautions are taken, marijuana smoking can gradually pervade all their waking hours. At that point, the habit is not easy to break.

Even the heaviest usage of marijuana does not lead to heroin or any other drug. Many junkies smoked marijuana before they tried opiates, but few marijuana users take narcotics. Many junkies also drank alcohol heavily, sometimes at very young ages, before they discovered heroin, yet no one argues that alcohol leads to heroin.

> The danger is this: over fifty percent of these young addicts started on marijuana smoking. They started there and graduated to heroin; they took up the needle when the thrill of marijuana was gone.
>
> — Federal Narcotics Commissioner Harry Anslinger in testimony to Congress in 1951

The reason, of course, is that alcohol enjoys general social approval, while marijuana is a "bad" drug and so invites false attributions of causality. Perhaps marijuana users are more likely than nonusers to try psychedelics and cocaine, because the distribution networks of these drugs overlap somewhat, but there is no quality of marijuana that induces its users to become consumers of other substances. The concept of marijuana as a "gateway drug" is nonsense.

Adaptation to marijuana enables users to learn to perform well under its influence. Unlike alcohol, it does not invariably depress reflexes and reaction times. People who aren't used to its effects will not be able to drive cars well or do any number of other routine tasks well while stoned. Even experienced users need time to practice a given task under the influence of marijuana in order to bring performance up to normal. Some users feel that marijuana helps them concentrate and enables them to work better, but even they have to learn to adapt to its effects. Most scientific tests show that marijuana impairs performance of all sorts. It is easy to come up with such results if you give marijuana to people who are not used to it, give it in much higher doses than they are used to, or give them hard tasks to perform, especially tasks that they have never done while stoned.

Many marijuana smokers drive cars, fly airplanes, ski, scuba dive, and engage in other hazardous activities after smoking. Many of them get away with it because they are experienced users with practice. This does not change the fact that marijuana can

> There have been a whole lot more people hurt on Astroturf
> than on grass.
> — Ken Kesey

drastically interfere with performance in some circumstances. Pot
and driving may not be as bad a combination for everyone as
drinking and driving, but it is certainly not a good one. For teen-
agers who drive recklessly to begin with, it is especially dangerous.

Proponents of marijuana like to argue its merits, trying to per-
suade others that it is really a beneficial drug. In fact, cannabis was
used in medicine in the past, and many doctors today feel that it is
still a valuable remedy for some ailments. Current federal laws
prohibit all uses of marijuana, but synthetic THC is available
(under the name Marinol), and many states have now legalized
marijuana for specific therapeutic uses. Unfortunately, federal law
takes precedence, and the federal government is waging an intense fight against medical marijuana.

Both THC and marijuana are good treatments for nausea and
vomiting. Doctors have used them successfully with cancer patients receiving chemotherapy, which involves very toxic drugs
that often cause intense stomach upset. This effect was first discovered by teen-agers with leukemia who happened to be pot
heads. Cannabis may also help asthma patients breathe easier, but
if it is smoked, the smoke will probably make them worse. It also
relaxes stiff muscles in a condition called spastic paralysis that results from brain injuries and diseases such as multiple sclerosis.
Finally, it stimulates appetite in wasting conditions that accom-
pany serious chronic diseases like AIDS and cancer. Conventional
medicine does not have good remedies for these conditions.

Although many patients prefer the effect of marijuana to that of
pure THC, federal agencies won't permit doctors to prescribe the
natural plant. Yet THC is not the same as whole marijuana and
may not be as safe. Recently, several pharmaceutical companies

I have multiple sclerosis. About three years after it was di-
agnosed, I discovered marijuana. A friend told me it was
relaxing. My main problem then, aside from partial blindness, was tenseness and tremors in my muscles. Pot cured
it, and I've smoked regularly ever since, about four to five
times a week. If I go without it for a week, the muscle tremors come back . . . Most people with MS have repeated
attacks and keep losing body function. I'm convinced that
pot has kept me in remission all these years.

— forty-one-year-old man, part-time roofer

have come up with synthetic drugs related to THC and have tried
to market them as antinausea remedies. In general, they are less
effective and more toxic than marijuana. The most recent development, from the United Kingdom, is a liquid whole-marijuana
preparation called Sativex, designed to be sprayed under the
tongue. It should be vastly superior to Marinol.

Aside from specific uses for serious medical problems, many
people find that pot relieves the symptoms of various mild ailments, from headaches to menstrual cramps. Probably, they use
the marijuana to get high and use the high as a way of taking their
mind off their discomfort. Taking your attention away from the
symptoms of a minor ailment sometimes will allow it to subside.
The less frequently you smoke marijuana, the more likely it is to
work for you as a medicine.

Of course, the same principle applies to getting high from pot.
The less frequently you use it, the better and more intense will be
your experiences with it. The main danger of smoking marijuana
is simply that it will get away from you, becoming more and more
of a repetitive habit and less and less of a useful way of changing
consciousness. The ease of integrating marijuana smoking with
all activities, from parties to sports to watching television, favors

habitual use. Also, tolerance for the interesting effects of the drug often encourages users to smoke more of it, when in fact they should be cutting down to increase their sensitivity. The absence of dramatic negative effects, such as a hangover, further encourages overuse. Unless you set rules for when and where you will smoke, you are likely to find yourself using pot more than you should — to the point where all the interesting and useful effects of the drug disappear and you are left with a stubborn, unproductive habit.

Some Suggestions About the Use of Marijuana

1. Marijuana is illegal. Being detected as a marijuana user (by urine screening or hair analysis, for example) can cost you your job and land you in a lot of trouble. Be aware of the dangers associated with acquiring an illegal drug. (See pages 204–205.)
2. Define what benefits you want from pot. Do not use it just because other people do or because it is available.
3. If you get effects that you like from marijuana, you will have to take precautions if you want to keep enjoying them.
4. Set limits on usage. For example, you may want to use pot only with certain friends, only on weekends, or only when you have no work to do. Such rules are necessary if you want to prevent your use from turning into a habit that gives you little satisfaction.
5. Remember that it can be dangerous to drive, operate machinery, or engage in hazardous activities under the influence of marijuana. The drug can cause illusions of time and space and always takes getting used to.
6. If you find the effects that you like from marijuana are becoming less intense or are disappearing altogether, *stop using it*. You can resume after a break and get them back. The trick is to keep frequency of use below the level where you become insensitive to marijuana's interesting effects on consciousness.

Odd as it may sound, less is more, and you can easily prove that to yourself.

7. If you find that the effects that you like are disappearing, the worst things you can do are smoke more or look for stronger pot. Those actions will just increase the problem.

8. Consider using marijuana by eating it in some form rather than smoking it. It is more trouble to take by mouth and the effects are different, but the risk of dependence is less. If you really prefer smoking, consider using a vaporizer.

9. Be careful about combining marijuana with other psychoactive drugs.

10. Be careful about set and setting, especially if you are trying marijuana for the first time.

11. Do not use marijuana on the job or at school. Most people would not drink alcohol in those situations, and just because it's easier to function on pot is no reason to use it. The more situations in which you allow yourself to smoke, the more likely you are to become dependent.

12. If you develop a cough or wheeze, or become more susceptible to chest colds, marijuana may be doing harm to your respiratory tract. Stop using it, cut down on use, or switch to eating it.

13. If you find that you are using marijuana more than you want to and are not getting useful effects from it, consider the possibility that it is controlling you more than you are controlling it. Try to do without it for a while. If you cannot, you may need outside help in breaking the habit.

14. If you have a medical condition that responds to marijuana, ask a doctor to write a letter supporting your use of it. In more and more places, local law-enforcement personnel will honor such letters, even if laws do not.

SUGGESTED READING

The best general history of marijuana is *Marihuana: The First Twelve Thousand Years* by Ernest L. Abel (London: Plenum, 1980). *Marijuana*

Botany by Robert Connell Clarke (second edition; Berkeley, Calif.: Ronin, 1992) is about the plant itself. It is lavishly illustrated. *Cannabis and Culture*, edited by Vera Rubin (The Hague, Netherlands: Mouton, 1975), is a fine collection of articles that looks at marijuana from various perspectives.

Marihuana Reconsidered by Lester Grinspoon, M.D. (second edition; Oakland, Calif.: Quick American Archives, 1994) is a comprehensive overview of the drug by a psychiatrist. *Cannabis and Cannabinoids: Pharmacology, Toxicology, and Therapeutic Potential*, edited by Franjo Grotenhermen, M.D., and Ethan Russo, M.D. (New York: Hawthorn Integrative Healing Press, 2002), is a comprehensive review of the pharmacology, botany, psychological effects, therapeutic potentials, and social and legal problems associated with both natural and synthetic cannabinoid compounds, with new and updated research from around the world.

The Marijuana Conviction: A History of Marijuana Prohibition in the United States by Richard J. Bonnie and Charles H. Whitebread (New York: Lindesmith Center, 1999) is a crisply written, scholarly history of marijuana in America. It discusses how the drug came to be classified as a dangerous narcotic and subjected to draconian laws.

Understanding Marijuana: A New Look at the Scientific Evidence by Mitch Earlywine (New York: Oxford University Press, 2002) is an excellent resource book and all-inclusive look at marijuana's history and pharmacology, its impact on thought and memory, the gateway effect, medical potentials, and law and policy.

In *The Emperor Wears No Clothes: The Authoritative Historical Record of the Cannabis Plant, Hemp Production, and How Marijuana Can Still Save the World* (Oakland, Calif.: Hemp Publishing, 1996), Jack Herer discusses how cannabis could provide the planet with an astonishing range of safe, nonpolluting products, from clothing to fuels.

Reefer Madness: Sex, Drugs, and Cheap Labor in the American Black Market by Eric Schlosser (New York: Mariner Books, 2003) is a highly detailed and comprehensive exploration of the causes and socioeconomic impact of the marijuana laws. It also looks at other facets of the underground economy in America. For a thoughtful historical analysis, see Jerome L. Himmelstein's *The Strange Career of Marihuana: Politics and the Ideology of Control in America* (Westport, Conn.: Greenwood, 1983).

Pot Planet: Adventures in Global Marijuana Culture by Brian Preston (New York: Grove Press, 2002) is an excellent firsthand account of a global trek to explore various marijuana cultures.

Louisa May Alcott wrote a short story about hashish in 1865 entitled "Perilous Play." A modern comic novel filled with references to marijuana is *The Fan Man* by William Kotzwinkle (reprint; New York: Vintage, 1994). Its hero, a delightful character named Horse Badorties, is never without pot. For a wonderful novel that tells the story of an eventful few months of growing marijuana in the backwoods of California, see T. Coraghessan Boyle's *Budding Prospects: A Pastoral* (reissue edition; New York: Viking, 1990).

Although teen-agers make up the bulk of the movie-going public, few films have capitalized on the popularity of marijuana among young people. Four older exceptions are *Up in Smoke* and *Nice Dreams* with Cheech and Chong; *The Harder They Come*, about marijuana in Jamaica in the 1970s; and Peter Fonda's classic from the 1960s, *Easy Rider*. An outrageous antimarijuana propaganda film from the 1930s, *Reefer Madness*, still plays on college campuses and in "art" movie houses, usually to the delight of mostly stoned audiences. Recent years have seen many poor marijuana movies, but two exceptions are *Dazed and Confused* and the documentary *Grass*, narrated by Woody Harrelson.

10. Solvents and Inhalants; Deliriants; PCP and Ketamine

THE DRUGS DESCRIBED in this chapter are a strange assortment of chemicals and plants that do not fit neatly into other categories. Some of them are more toxic than the substances discussed earlier, and, though all of them have their devoted fans, experienced users regard them as second-rate or substitute drugs, not worth taking unless preferred drugs are unavailable.

Organic Solvents

In chemistry, the word *organic* refers to compounds of carbon. Some of the simplest organic chemicals are clear, volatile liquids made by distilling petroleum. These liquids have many uses in industry. Some, like gasoline, make good fuels because they burn readily. Others, like benzene and toluene, dissolve grease and oil, making them useful as cleaning fluids and solvents.

The fumes of these organic solvents have strong chemical odors and make people feel lightheaded, hot, and dizzy. Cans and bottles of them usually carry warning labels about using them only with good ventilation. Many people dislike breathing solvent fumes, but some find it interesting and repeatedly sniff certain household products or gasoline to change their state of consciousness. Products containing organic solvents include some glues (rubber cement and model airplane glue), paint thinner, lighter fluid, and varnish, wax, and spot removers.

TAJAR: What made you want to smell gas, Bullet?

BULLET: Well, when you feel bad, you smell it and it makes you feel kind of hot and kind of drowsy, like you was floating through the air. It makes you feel sort of hot inside and different from the way you were before . . .

TAJAR: Bullet, how come so much gas was spilled on the cellar floor?

BULLET: Oh, I just wanted to get more on my rag. If you have a lot it makes you sort of dream. It gets all dark and you see shooting stars in it, and this time I saw big flies flying in it. They were big and green and had white wings.

— from an interview with a young gasoline sniffer, quoted in *Licit and Illicit Drugs,* by Edward M. Brecher and the editors of *Consumer Reports* (1972)

As psychoactive drugs, the organic solvents produce effects resembling low doses of general anesthetic, but they are more toxic and tend to cause dizziness, nausea, and other uncomfortable physical feelings. In high doses, they may induce visual hallucinations and vivid waking dreams. Some young people find that the effects are similar to the dizzy excitement that comes from spinning around. Since many children use spinning as a technique for changing their awareness, and since organic solvents are commonly found around the house, many children come to experiment with them. Often, these chemicals are a child's first introduction to consciousness-change by means of drugs.

Children who regularly sniff solvents develop tolerance for them. Although there is no physical withdrawal as with alcohol and narcotics, the sniffing habit can be very difficult to break. Just like grown-up drunks, solvent-sniffing children may spend most of their waking time in a stupor, unable to do their work or pay attention to what really matters.

Probably, some people have sniffed solvents occasionally over the years, just as some people have played with chloroform, ether, and nitrous oxide. For the most part, this use never attracted much notice. Beginning about 1959, however, newspapers in the United States began to focus attention on glue-sniffing as a new drug menace spreading among children in cities of the West and Midwest. A few children died from lack of oxygen by putting glue in plastic bags, then putting the bags over their heads. Seizing upon these cases, newspapers dramatized the hazards of glue-sniffing, making it seem extremely dangerous. Parents' groups and police officials then called for laws against it. The main effect of all this attention was to stimulate curiosity about glue-sniffing and cause a tremendous increase in the number of people doing it. At the beginning of the 1960s, gasoline sniffing was the most popular form of organic solvent use. Sniffing of other substances was rare and caused no concern. Then came a hysterical nation-wide crusade against glue-sniffing with scare stories in newspapers, legislative hearings, and, finally, arrest and imprisonment of some children. Only glue-sniffing received this kind of attention, and only glue-sniffing became enormously popular. Today, significant numbers of schoolchildren have tried or used glue in an attempt to get high.

All of the scare stories exaggerated the dangers of solvent inhalation, saying that it certainly led to brain, heart, and liver damage, destruction of the bone marrow, blindness, and death. There *is* medical evidence of harm from exposure to organic solvents, but most of it concerns factory workers who breathe the fumes all day long over months and years or rare individuals who drink the liquids. Young people who sniff solvents occasionally are not likely to develop these serious medical problems.

As with alcohol, anesthetics, and the other depressants, use of solvents can produce disorientation and impairment of judgment and coordination. Since these changes favor accidents, it would be silly to sniff solvent fumes while driving or doing anything else requiring good reflexes. Overdoses of fumes may lead to unconsciousness, and with complete lack of oxygen, death is a real possibility. Also, it is unwise to mix sniffing with drinking, both because that combination puts a great deal of stress on the liver and because it can depress respiration to a dangerous degree. In pregnant women, solvent fumes may raise the risk of birth defects. Fumes of some of the solvents can irritate the membranes of the nose.

Inhalation puts these chemicals into the blood and brain very fast, so the effects come on almost immediately. They usually last from fifteen minutes to half an hour after sniffing stops. Some people breathe fumes directly from the container; others put solvents or glue on a rag or in a paper bag. The practice is usually called "huffing" or "bagging."

The majority of huffers are between the ages of ten and seventeen, with children of certain ethnic groups predominating. The most common sniffers have been Hispanic males. Many Native American boys also sniff solvents — a source of great concern on many Indian reservations. African-American children, on the other hand, seem to prefer other drugs, and, until recently, few girls used solvents. No one knows why these differences exist, and today, with rising use of all drugs among young people, the older patterns may be changing.

Grown-ups tend to regard glue, gasoline, paint thinner, and the rest as cheap highs — easy to obtain and not very good. Among people who have tried many drugs, the organic solvents are always considered low class and second rate, much inferior to drugs such as alcohol and marijuana. The popularity of solvents among children reflects their easy availability and dramatic power to change consciousness fast rather than any really desirable qualities about them. When children grow up and discover other drugs that are less toxic and more useful, they generally stop playing around with solvents.

Aerosol Propellants

Until recently, most aerosol products contained types of fluorocarbons known by the brand name Freon. Freon, when inhaled, produces the same effects as the organic solvents and presents the same risks to the user. Because scientists now recognize that fluorocarbons damage the earth's atmosphere, manufacturers have switched to other propellants, usually simpler organic compounds that also cause changes in consciousness when people inhale them.

Inhaling aerosol propellants is a bit more complicated than inhaling solvents because the propellants come mixed with other substances. For example, when you press the button on a can of black spray paint, what comes out is a cloud of tiny droplets of black paint and gas. Inhaling black paint does not get you high and can make you very sick. Some users solve this problem by spraying the can into a bag or balloon so that the particles separate from the gas by adhering to the sides. Others turn the cans upside down so that only the propellant comes out, and still others inhale the sprays through cloth filters.

Nitrite Inhalants

Amyl Nitrite (Amys, Poppers, Snappers, Pearls, Aspirol, Vaporal)

Amyl nitrite is a simple chemical that has been used for more than a hundred years to relieve heart pain in people who suffer from coronary artery disease. Such people often feel severe chest pain when they exert themselves. If they breathe the fumes of amyl nitrite, the pain quickly disappears because the drug dilates arteries throughout the body, reducing the workload of the heart. Other effects are a sudden fall in blood pressure, a throbbing feeling in the head (or even a brief pounding headache), occasional dizziness and nausea, warmth and flushing of the skin, and a dramatically altered state of consciousness that reminds some people of fainting or going under general anesthesia.

Amyl nitrite is a clear, yellowish liquid with a strong chemical smell. It comes in inhalers and in cloth-covered glass capsules that can be crushed in the hand and sniffed. (They break with an audible "pop" — hence the common street name *poppers*.) Until 1960, amyl nitrite was a prescription drug. Although some people used it recreationally, most buyers were heart patients who carried it with them for medical purposes and did not think of it as a mind-changing substance. Then the Food and Drug Administration removed the prescription requirement, so that amyl nitrite became an over-the-counter drug, available to anyone.

During the 1960s, many users of street drugs experimented with amyl nitrite as a quick, legal high. It appealed especially to young people, to those who liked to sniff organic solvents, and to those who liked the highs of general anesthetics. In addition, poppers had a special reputation as an enhancer of sexual experience. Inhaled during a sexual act, the drug is supposed to intensify the experience and prolong and intensify orgasm. Although some heterosexual men and women use it in this way, male homosexuals have been the greatest fans of amyl nitrite. The effects of a single, deep inhalation last only for a few minutes and are often followed by less pleasant sensations, but gay men may pass the drug back and forth many times while having sex.

As recreational use of amyl nitrite spread, authorities opposed its unrestricted sale. Finally, in 1969, the Food and Drug Administration reimposed the prescription requirement, ending over-the-counter distribution. Today, however, it is still in wide use, especially in the gay community.

All nitrites are poisonous in excess, but amyl nitrite, when inhaled, breaks down easily and leaves the body very quickly. It is considered one of the safest drugs in medicine, and even people who inhale it frequently do not seem to suffer ill effects. Still, it is probably not wise to overdo it. The strong chemical odor of amyl nitrite is suggestive of materials that are hard on the body; it is possible that long-term use has physical consequences that doctors do not yet recognize. It should not be used at all by people with anemia, glaucoma, high blood pressure, or a recent head injury. Also, it may be harmful to pregnant women. Because the liquid drug can corrode the cornea, users should be careful to keep it away from their eyes.

Because amyl nitrite causes a sudden drop in blood pressure, it

> I was first introduced to amyl nitrite during my senior year
> in college. The father of one of my friends had a heart con-
> dition for which he used the drug. He would amass huge
> numbers of poppers and give them out to anyone who
> wanted them ... The effect was immediate. My arms and
> legs felt like liquid warmth, and at the same time, I got
> a pounding in my head ... When I exhaled, my vision
> blurred, with small blue patches filling my field of vision.
>
> — twenty-year-old man, medical student

can produce loss of coordination and fainting. It should not be inhaled in situations requiring muscular coordination or careful
posture. Also, it should be used with good ventilation and never be
put into closed containers, such as plastic bags, for continuous
breathing. As with organic solvents, that method can lead to suffo-
cation.

Butyl Nitrite and Isobutyl Nitrite (Locker Room, Rush)

Butyl nitrite and isobutyl nitrite are close chemical relatives of
amyl nitrite that were not under any drug regulations for a long
time. They used to be sold by mail order and over the counter in
head shops. They came in small bottles or aerosol cans with labels
identifying them as "liquid incense" or "room odorizer," but everyone who bought these products knew what they were for. Butyl
nitrite and isobutyl nitrite are now banned. Their effects are the
same as those of poppers.

Some Precautions About Organic Solvents and Inhalants

1. Organic solvents are highly flammable. Never use them near
   open flames or sparks.

2. People have died of asphyxiation by putting their heads in plastic bags containing small amounts of solvents.

3. Never sniff solvents while driving, operating machinery, or engaging in other hazardous activities requiring good reflexes, coordination, and attention.

4. If you sniff solvents, get plenty of fresh air afterward to flush the chemical out of your system.

5. Do not sniff solvents while drinking alcohol or using other depressants.

6. Do not sniff solvents if you have a history of liver disease.

7. Regular sniffing of solvents can become a stubborn drug habit, much like alcoholism. If you develop this pattern of use, you may need outside help to break it.

8. Remember that people who are most experienced with psychoactive drugs always say that highs from organic solvents are second rate.

9. Amyl, butyl, and isobutyl nitrite are less toxic than organic solvents and not as flammable. They should be used only with good ventilation and not breathed continuously.

10. Inhale nitrites only when you are in a comfortable sitting or lying position.

11. Be careful not to get liquid nitrites in your eyes.

Deliriants

Delirium is a state of mental disturbance marked by confusion and disorientation. People in delirium cannot think clearly and may not remember who they are, where they are, or what year it is. They may also hallucinate, seeing and hearing things that are not there. Usually, delirium is a temporary condition resulting from some disorder of the brain. For example, a high fever will cause delirium; when the fever comes down, the delirium ends. If you can remember the experience of a high fever as a young child, you know what delirium is.

Overdose of most psychoactive drugs will cause delirium because they are temporarily toxic to the brain. This kind of delirium is called a toxic psychosis because it is a malfunction of the brain that results from the presence of a toxin in the body. As the drug overdose is metabolized and eliminated, the toxic psychosis resolves. If delirium is very strong, people may not remember it clearly afterward, that is, they may have some degree of amnesia for the experience.

Depending on what causes the delirium, there may be physical effects as well, usually uncomfortable ones such as nausea, dizziness, headache, and prostration. The mental experiences are variable, too, and although many people find them unpleasant, some find them powerfully fascinating, more vivid than ordinary reality. Here is one man's description of a visual hallucination he had as a child during a high fever:

"I was standing on a cliff looking down at an ocean of cream. Somehow I knew that the cream was just about to curdle, and there was something absolutely horrible about that. But the tension just kept building and building. The ocean of cream was always just on the point of curdling, and the tension was unbearable. It is one of the most vivid memories of my childhood."

Some drugs, called deliriants, cause delirium at subtoxic doses. They come from chemicals found in a strange group of plants, some of which have been used for thousands of years to induce altered states of consciousness. Deliriants certainly do not appeal to all people, and some of them are dangerous. Nevertheless, they remain popular.

Nightshades (Jimsonweed, Datura, Belladonna, Henbane)

The nightshade family of plants includes some very popular foods: tomatoes, sweet and hot peppers, eggplant, and potatoes. It also includes tobacco and some poisonous plants that are infamous because of their association with crime, witchcraft, and black magic. Even their names are sinister: henbane, mandrake, and deadly nightshade, for example. Nightshades look scary, too.

They are rank, hairy plants with strange smells and peculiar flowers; some have dangerous fruit.

In North America, the main poisonous nightshades are two species of datura: *Datum stramonium,* or jimsonweed, in the East and *Datura meteloides,* or sacred datura, in the West. Sacred datura is so called because of its long involvement with Native American magic and religion.

All parts of these plants contain scopolamine, a drug that causes delirium and can be seriously poisonous in high doses. The lowest concentration of scopolamine is in the roots, making them the safest part of the plant to consume. The highest concentrations are in the seeds, making them the most dangerous. Roots, seeds, leaves, and flowers can all be eaten, smoked, brewed into teas, or even ground up in fat and rubbed on the skin. All of these methods put scopolamine into the bloodstream and cause intoxication.

The physical effects of scopolamine are very dramatic and often very uncomfortable. They include parched mouth and burning thirst; hot, dry skin and a feverish feeling; widely dilated eyes (making bright light painful); inability to focus the eyes at close distances; rapid heart rate; constipation; difficulty in urinating; and, in men, interference with ejaculation. These effects may last for twelve to forty-eight hours after a single dose of datura.

The mental effects are equally dramatic: restlessness, disorientation, and other symptoms of delirium, including vivid hallucinations that may seem so real that people lose all contact with ordinary reality. Because scopolamine usually leaves you with some amnesia, it is often hard to remember these hallucinations clearly when the drug wears off. Going into other worlds is fascinating, but the worlds that datura takes people to can be frightening, populated by monsters and devils and filled with violent, frenzied energy.

The ability of plants containing scopolamine to disconnect people from ordinary reality accounts for their popularity in certain circles. Criminals have used them for centuries in all parts of the world, slipping them to unsuspecting victims to make it easier to rob, rape, or kidnap them. Witches in medieval Europe used deadly nightshade (belladonna), henbane, and mandrake to have the experience of flying and to meet the devil in their visions. American Indian medicine men have used jimsonweed and sacred datura to initiate young men into the mysteries of the spirit world and to seek visions in group religious rituals.

Today, datura seems to appeal mostly to young people seeking strong intoxication. The plant is easily available in many places and is very powerful. It is in wide use as a recreational drug, often in combination with alcohol, among teen-agers on Indian reservations in the West. Drug crisis centers throughout the United States see frequent cases of bad trips on datura.

Although medical doctors consider datura very dangerous, it will probably not do physical harm to the average healthy person. The main danger of datura is accidental death or injury resulting from disorientation. For example, people intoxicated on this plant have drowned by stumbling into deep bodies of water, perhaps in an effort to quench the thirst and fever caused by scopolamine. Others, experiencing monsters chasing them, have taken serious falls.

Scopolamine is still used as a medical drug. Low doses can be applied to the skin in special patches to prevent motion sickness. Until recently, it also went into over-the-counter sleeping pills as well as some cold and allergy tablets to dry up a runny nose. Higher doses used to be given by injection to women in labor ("twilight sleep") to make them amnesic for the experience of childbirth, a practice that was not beneficial to either mother or baby because it produced a predictable, violent delirium. At one time, jimsonweed leaves were rolled into cigarettes for the treatment of asthma, and tincture of belladonna is still occasionally used to treat gastrointestinal spasms.

Amanita Mushrooms (Fly Agaric, Amanita muscaria; Panther Mushroom, Amanita pantherina)

Amanitas are a family of large, beautiful mushrooms that grow in many parts of the world. Some of them are deadly, the most poisonous of all wild mushrooms. Some are edible and delicious. Two are neither deadly nor edible as food but are used as psychoactive drugs.

Amanita muscaria, the fly agaric, is a big mushroom with white dots on a red or orange cap. (*Agaric* is an old word for mushroom; the name *fly* comes from an old practice of chopping this mushroom into a saucer of milk to attract and kill flies.) The fly agaric is often pictured in illustrations of fairy tales and cannot be mistaken for any other mushroom. Fly agarics growing in the eastern United States are yellow and not usually psychoactive. Those in the western states are red or orange; their pharmacological power correlates with cap color, the reddest mushrooms being strongest.

Amanita muscaria was the traditional intoxicant of a number of primitive tribes of Siberia — people who did not have access to other drugs but did have a shamanistic religion similar to that of many Native Americans. In the 1960s, news stories about the intoxicating effect of this mushroom led many young people in California and other western states to experiment with it as a new natural high.

People have consumed the fly agaric in many forms. The red peel of the cap, which is easily removed, can be dried and smoked. The whole mushroom can be eaten fresh, cooked, or dried, or it can be brewed into a tea and drunk. These different preparations may produce different results. Also, the mushrooms seem to vary greatly in strength and effect, depending on where and when they grow and what trees they grow around.

Moderate doses cause a dreamy intoxication that some people find pleasant, but there are often uncomfortable physical symptoms. High doses can produce delirious excitement and significant toxicity. The effect comes on within thirty minutes and lasts for four to eight hours.

The chemicals responsible are ibotenic acid and muscimol, substances that resemble GABA, one of the brain's own neurotransmitters. Higher doses of them are found in a close relative of *Amanita muscaria,* a brown mushroom with white dots called the panther mushroom, or *Amanita pantherina*. It grows in woods in the Pacific Northwest and other parts of the world, and in recent years many people have also experimented with it as a way of altering their consciousness.

Again, the panther's effects are very variable, so that it may be hard to estimate a manageable dose and easy to take too much. High doses of the panther can make people very sick for up to twelve hours, and a few eaters of it have injured themselves as a result of accidents while they were delirious.

It would be foolish to experiment with either of these mushrooms without good advice from someone experienced with them about exact dose and method of preparation.

Nutmeg and Mace

Nutmeg, the ground spice that goes into cookies, eggnog, and pumpkin pie, contains a drug called myristicin that may be converted in the body to one of the amphetamine-like psychedelics. Nutmeg is the seed of a tropical tree. The outer covering of this seed is ground into a similar spice, called mace, that often flavors cakes. Both nutmeg and mace have a long history of use as psychoactive drugs, especially by people who can't obtain better ones.

To get high on nutmeg or mace, you have to eat a lot of them:

Someone told me you could get high by eating nutmeg. So one night I choked down a whole can, which was over an ounce. After three hours, I felt light and dreamy. It was a little like a light dose of pot. However, the next morning, I had a splitting headache, my heart was racing, and my mouth was really dry. I got dizzy whenever I managed to stand up. It lasted all day. I would never eat nutmeg again. I don't even like the taste of it in food anymore.

— twenty-two-year-old man, carpenter

from a tablespoon up to a whole spice-can full. In that quantity, these spices taste awful. They are also fairly toxic and regularly leave people with a heavy hangover the next day. The effects are variable, ranging from mild feelings of floating to full-blown delirium. Most people who try nutmeg out of curiosity do not come back for a second try. Frequent users are usually found only in certain prisons or other situations where more desirable drugs are unobtainable.

Some Warnings About Deliriants

1. Delirium is an abnormal condition of the brain in which mental function is temporarily deranged. A delirious person doing anything other than lying still in a safe place is a good candidate for a serious accident.
2. Never take deliriant drugs by yourself. Make sure someone not under the influence of the drug is there to watch out for you.
3. If you must experiment with jimsonweed or other nightshades, use the root rather than leaves or seeds.
4. Do not experiment with *Amanita muscaria* or *Amanita pantherina* without good advice about dose and preparation from an experienced person in the area where the mushrooms grow. Smoking the dried colored peel of these mushrooms is the mildest way of taking them.
5. If you eat nutmeg or mace in an effort to get high, be prepared for a terrific hangover the next day.

PCP and Ketamine

The last two drugs in this chapter are strange synthetic compounds different from any other drugs. They are often called anesthetics, but unlike the general anesthetics discussed in Chapter 7, they are not depressants. In fact, they stimulate the vital functions of heartbeat and respiration, even though they produce some mental effects resembling anesthesia. Other people call them psychedelics, but they are very different from those drugs, too.

PCP (Angel Dust, Peace Pill, Hog, Animal Tranquilizer, "THC," "Cannabinol")

PCP (phencyclidine) was invented in a pharmaceutical laboratory in the late 1950s and was introduced into clinical medicine in the United States in 1963 under the trade name Sernyl. It was marketed as a surgical anesthetic but did not make people unconscious in the same way as ether. Rather, it "dissociated" consciousness from the body so that patients were not bothered by surgical procedures even though they retained some kind of awareness. Enthusiasm about the medical value of PCP diminished when reports began to come in of unpleasant side effects in many patients. These reactions included strange mental states, such as feelings of being out of the body, and visual disturbances that some patients found frightening. In 1965, the drug was withdrawn from use for humans, but two years later it was reintroduced as a veterinary anesthetic under the name Sernylan. Animals could not tell their veterinarians that they disliked the side effects.

Shortly thereafter, PCP appeared on the black market. It is a cheap and easy drug to make, produces a strong intoxication, and can be sold to unsuspecting buyers as other, more desirable drugs. For instance, pills of PCP have often been sold as synthetic THC, the chief component of marijuana. (In fact, synthetic THC is very rare and expensive and is almost never available on the black market.) Supermarket mushrooms, treated with PCP alone or with PCP and LSD, were sold as magic mushrooms throughout the late 1960s and early 1970s. PCP-LSD combinations have also been sold as mescaline and psilocybin.

PCP comes as both pills and a powder. The powdered form, called angel dust, can be sprinkled in a joint made of marijuana or inactive herbs such as parsley, mint, and oregano, or it can be dissolved in an organic solvent and sprayed on these materials. When the solvent evaporates, it leaves an even residue of the drug.

Such joints are called dusters. Some people snort angel dust, and very few inject it. By any route, PCP produces distinctive effects. It causes decreased sensitivity to pain and a peculiar rubbery feeling in the legs with impaired coordination. It may also cause dizziness and nausea, flushing, sweating, and abnormal movements of the eyes.

The mental effects are very variable but often include a feeling of disconnection from the body and from external reality, apathy, disorganization of thinking, a drunklike state, and distortions of time and space perception. Overdoses can cause convulsions and coma. When it is smoked, PCP's effects come on within a few minutes, peak within five to thirty minutes, and last for four to six hours. Oral doses may last longer, and some people say they do not feel normal for up to twenty-four hours after a single oral dose.

Throughout the 1960s and early 1970s, most people who took PCP took it unwittingly, thinking that they were taking something else — mescaline, psilocybin, or some sort of supermarijuana. It came in all kinds of disguises. Few people took it for its own merits, and it had an unsavory reputation, often disparaged as an "animal tranquilizer."

In more recent years, however, PCP has become even more prevalent, and some people seek it out as their drug of choice. The PCP lovers who have received the most publicity are teen-agers from urban ghettos whose lives are filled with anger, frustration, and violence. Maybe they like the feeling of being cut off from the grim reality of their environment or from their own emotions. Because of heavy use of PCP by such persons, the drug has now gained a reputation for causing crime, violence, and insanity among young people. No doubt, some PCP-related murders have occurred, but newspapers, predictably, have blown the drug's association with violence out of all proportion, leading to legislative hearings and stiffer laws on PCP, as well as great hysteria about a new drug menace.

There does not seem to be anything about the pharmacology of PCP that automatically makes users become violent or commit

I've had very positive experiences with PCP, which is unusual, since everyone says it's a terrible drug . . . For years I have suffered lower back pains. Whenever I smoked PCP, I felt no pain and could even jog comfortably. Even after the drug wore off, I experienced no pain from physical activities . . . My thinking was often imaginative and lucid. I laughed a lot . . . I was taking it all the time, and people around me told me I was acting too crazily. So I stopped. Sometime I'd like to experiment with it again to explore those physical and mental powers it seems to release in me.

— thirty-six-year-old man, screenwriter

crime. Clearly, high doses can make people agitated and confused, but tendencies to criminal violence are inherent in certain people, not in certain drugs. PCP users who are not angry and violent to begin with do not become raving lunatics after smoking angel dust. The rash of scare stories about PCP seems to reflect society's need to have "devil drugs" more than it does the nature of PCP.

The main arguments against PCP are that its effects seem neither very interesting nor very productive for most people. Some users take it in ways that they find valuable — for example, as a social or party drug much like alcohol and downers — but many young persons take it just to get "messed up" or feel disconnected from reality. Also, the adulteration of other drugs with PCP is a deplorable practice, especially when these are sold or given to unsuspecting people.

Adverse reactions to PCP can include inability to talk or communicate, a blank stare and robotlike attitude, rigid muscles, confusion, agitation, and paranoid thinking. Heavy users sometimes develop problems with speech and memory that may last for some time after they stop taking the drug.

Ketamine (Ketalar, Ketaject, Super-K, Vitamin K)

Ketamine is a close relative of PCP, producing very similar effects. It is a legal prescription drug intended for use as an anesthetic. Ketamine comes in small bottles as a solution to be injected, either intravenously or intramuscularly.

Like PCP, ketamine produces an unusual kind of anesthesia, called a dissociative state, in which the patient's awareness becomes detached from the body and from external reality. Like PCP, ketamine has produced a number of bad reactions, since many patients become frightened when they find themselves in this unusual condition. So far, however, there has been no move to take ketamine off the market.

In recent years, a number of people have experimented with ketamine as a recreational drug, but they have been very different from PCP users, with the result that ketamine has a very different reputation and following from its notorious relative.

In the first place, all ketamine is manufactured legally. Since it is not a controlled substance, it is not closely watched, and supplies of it are easily diverted from hospitals and pharmacies into the hands of recreational users. Many of its fans are doctors who have introduced their friends, including nurses and other professionals, to the drug. Ketamine users tend to be better educated, older, wealthier, and much more experienced with drugs than most PCP users. They are able to take exact doses of pure material.

Because ketamine comes in an injectable form and because many of its users are medical personnel, it tends to be taken by injection, usually intramuscularly. Given in this way, it produces an altered state of consciousness that begins in a few minutes and lasts about half an hour. The feeling is one of dreamy, floating disconnection from external reality. Some ketamine enthusiasts like to take it while lying in a sensory isolation tank in an attempt to have an out-of-body experience.

The fact that ketamine remained an uncontrolled substance while PCP came to be seen as the chief devil drug of the 1980s is a good illustration of how the image of a drug is shaped by its users. Just as marijuana has never shaken off its association with deviants, minorities, and rebels, so PCP is now linked with an angry, violent, young segment of the population that is prone to commit crime. PCP does not cause crime, violence, or insanity any more than marijuana causes revolutions. The pharmacology of ketamine is practically the same as that of PCP, yet ketamine users (usually successful professionals) lie peacefully in dissociative states, causing no one any harm, and raising few alarms in society.

Unfortunately, many ketamine users do not realize that they can take the drug by safer routes than injection. Ketamine liquid can be evaporated to solid crystals that can be powdered and smoked, snorted, or swallowed, just like PCP. By the oral route, ketamine lasts longer, and the peak effect is less dramatic. By any route, high doses of ketamine can be as unpleasant as high doses of PCP.

Some Suggestions About PCP and Ketamine

1. Try to avoid taking PCP unintentionally. All street psychedelics in pill or powder form are suspect, as are funny-tasting joints that give a strange rush.
2. If you take PCP deliberately, avoid high doses.
3. As with other drugs, the oral route is safer. Smoking PCP gives a rapid, dramatic effect. Some users prefer to smoke it, because they know right away how high they are. If you take PCP by mouth, it is even more important to know the dose so that you don't get more intoxicated than you intend.
4. Do not take PCP with depressants or stimulants. The combined effects can be unpleasant and difficult to control.
5. Because PCP affects coordination, thought, and judgment, do

not do things under its influence that require those functions to be normal.

6. Because PCP can produce agitation, confusion, and difficulties in communication, it is not wise to take it in settings or with people that might add to those problems.

7. If you take PCP regularly and find you have trouble thinking clearly or remembering, cut down or stop taking it altogether.

8. If you meet people who want you to try ketamine, remember that it is essentially the same as PCP.

9. Remember also that ketamine can be taken by mouth and does not have to be injected.

SUGGESTED READING

Very few good books on solvent abuse are in print, and most of the available literature is aimed at a younger audience than our readers. A good book on the dangers of inhalants for teen-agers is *Need to Know: Solvent Abuse* by Sean Connolly (Portsmouth, N.H.: Heinemann Educational, 2002). A good Web site for information on solvents (and many other drugs) is The Vault of Erowid, www.erowid.org (last accessed April 2004).

For information on nightshade plants, see *The Fascinating World of the Nightshades: Tobacco, Mandrake, Potato, Tomato, Pepper, Eggplant, Etc.* by Charles Bixler Heiser (Mineola, N.Y.: Dover, 1987). The book discusses the edible nightshades and tobacco as well as the deliriant members of the family. For more on other psychoactive herbs, see *Legal Highs: A Concise Encyclopedia of Legal Herbs & Chemicals with Psychoactive Properties* by Adam Gottlieb (Berkeley, Calif.: Ronin, 1991).

Jonathan Ott includes *Amanita muscaria* and *Amanita pantherina* in his *Hallucinogenic Plants of North America* (reprint; New York: Bantam, 1993). In *Mushrooms and Mankind: The Impact of Mushrooms on Human Consciousness and Religion* (Escondido, Calif.: Book Tree, 2000), James Arthur tries to link many of the world's religions with Amanita cults.

A good book about ketamine is *Ketamine: Dreams and Realities* by Karl Jansen, M.D. (Sarasota, Fla.: Multidisciplinary Association for Psychedelic Studies (MAPS), 2001).

11. Medical Drugs; Herbal Remedies; Smart Drugs

A GREAT MANY psychoactive drugs are sold legally: as prescription medicines used by doctors, as over-the-counter remedies stocked in drugstores, and as herbal products available in many health food stores. Patients and consumers are often unaware of the effects of these substances. We review the more common ones in this chapter.

Psychiatric Drugs

Psychiatrists now rely heavily on drugs to treat the symptoms of mental illness. Although these chemicals do affect mood, perception, and thought, they rarely cause euphoria or trigger high states; as a result, people generally do not take them unless they are psychiatric patients. Psychiatric medications fall into four main categories: antipsychotics, antidepressants, antimanic drugs, and antianxiety agents. We discussed the last of these in Chapter 7.

Antipsychotic Drugs (Major Tranquilizers)

Major tranquilizers revolutionized psychiatry when they were first introduced in the early 1950s. They provided a new and easy way to manage schizophrenia and other severe mental diseases, making patients calm and emotionally quiet. In some cases, the major tranquilizers have enabled psychotic persons to lead rea-

> I firmly believe that if the whole materia medica as now used could be sunk to the bottom of the sea, it would be all the better for mankind and all the worse for the fishes.
>
> — Oliver Wendell Holmes (1809–1894), American physician and author

sonably normal lives and function outside hospitals. More often, tranquilizers make these people more manageable and docile rather than less crazy.

The most widely used drug in this group was chlorpromazine (Thorazine). It belongs to a group of drugs called phenothiazines that also include prochlorperazine (Compazine) and trifluoperazine (Stelazine). In addition to their use in treating mental illness, the phenothiazines can be used to end bad reactions to psychedelic drugs and other states of confusion. Some of them are also used to treat purely physical problems, such as itching, dizziness, nausea, vomiting, and hiccups.

In normal people, small doses of these compounds cause drowsiness, lethargy, and boredom — hardly the kinds of effects that encourage recreational use. In addition, the major tranquilizers regularly produce uncomfortable physical effects, such as dryness of the mouth. In high doses and long-term use, they can also cause more serious toxicity, such as liver and eye damage and permanent disorders of muscle movement and coordination.

Newer types of antipsychotic drugs are now in wide use, such as haloperidol (Haldol), risperidone (Risperdal), and clozapine (Clozaril). They are more effective than phenothiazines for some schizophrenic patients, but all have the potential to cause serious toxicity.

Because the physical and mental effects of antipsychotic drugs are at best uninteresting and at worst very unpleasant, nonmedical use of them is nonexistent.

Antidepressants (Tricyclics and SSRIs)

The word *antidepressant* sounds attractive. It suggests a drug that lifts your mood and makes you feel good, something like a stimulant. The antidepressant drugs used in psychiatry today, however, do not give the good feelings of stimulants. Instead, they often cause sedation and a variety of uncomfortable physical effects.

These drugs date from 1958, when the parent compound, imipramine (Tofranil), was invented. It is still in use today, along with a close relative, amitriptyline (Elavil), and a number of other similar drugs, called tricyclics for their chemical structure. Some depressed patients respond very well to these medications but not until after at least two weeks of regular use. On the other hand, the toxic effects begin right away: sedation, dry mouth, blurred vision, constipation, difficulty in urinating. Normal people are likely to notice only these "side effects" without any positive mood changes.

A newer class of antidepressant drugs is the selective serotonin reuptake inhibitors, or SSRIs; the first to appear was fluoxetine (Prozac). It was followed by sertraline (Zoloft), paroxetine (Paxil), and citalopram (Celexa), all of which have become extremely popular medical drugs. SSRIs can produce different side effects from the tricyclics: anxiety, impotence in men, and suicidal thinking, for example. Some commentators complain that widespread prescription of SSRIs has made many Americans less interesting and less creative.

One anomalous antidepressant drug is bupropion (Wellbutrin), also marketed as an aid to smoking cessation under the brand name Zyban. Unlike the other compounds discussed here, it is a stimulant of the central nervous system, and some users of stimulants may like that effect. Bupropion also commonly causes anxiety and jitteriness and, in high doses, seizures.

Like the major tranquilizers, the antidepressants do not lend themselves to recreational use because few people like their immediate effects. Often, even depressed patients who are helped by them like to cut their dosage to a minimum and do without them altogether when they can. Do not be misled by their name: antidepressants will not make you high.

Drugs for Treating Bipolar Disorder

Manic-depressive psychosis, also known as bipolar disorder, is a serious mental illness in which people swing back and forth between extremes of mood, from intense elation (mania) to intense depression. There is a high risk of suicide in these patients. An older drug used to treat bipolar disorder is lithium carbonate (Ekalith), which evens out the mood swings and is especially good at preventing manic episodes, although it is also used to treat depression. It has many side effects and can produce serious toxicity in the nervous system, heart, and kidneys. A newer drug is divalproex sodium (Depakote), also with a significant potential for toxicity. Neither of these drugs has any effect on the mind that would recommend them for nonmedical use.

Prescription Drugs Not Commonly Thought to Be Psychoactive

Many medical drugs have mental effects that are ignored by doctors who prescribe them. Often, these effects are listed as "side effects" in the fine-print information that manufacturers include with drugs. Sometimes, patients find the side effects more prominent than the main effects.

Antihistamines

Some allergic reactions are mediated by an endogenous substance called histamine that strongly affects nerves, blood vessels, and other tissues. In an effort to suppress allergic symptoms, pharmacologists have invented a number of synthetic drugs to

Throughout junior high school and high school, I suffered from bad hay fever. My family doctor prescribed antihistamines for me. They definitely worked, but they made me feel so bad. Finally, I came to prefer the hay fever. I was happier sneezing than being so depressed and logy. Once, while in college, I took a twenty-five-milligram tablet of Thorazine and I was amazed at how similar the effect was to the antihistamines. I hate that feeling. I managed to get rid of most of my allergies by changing my diet and lifestyle. I haven't taken an antihistamine in years.

— thirty-eight-year-old man, musician

block the actions of histamine. Many antihistamines are now available; in large-dosage forms, they are dispensed by prescription, but lower-dosage forms are sold over the counter. Some of the ones in widespread use are diphenhydramine (Benadryl), chlorpheniramine (Teldrin, Chlor-Trimeton), brompheniramine (Dimetane), dexchlorpheniramine (Polaramine), tripelennamine (PBZ, Pyribenzamine), tripolidine (Actidil), promethazine (Phenergan), pyrilamine, and doxylamine.

Although antihistamines are strong drugs that affect many systems of the body, they are often not very efficient at doing what they are supposed to do: counteract histamine and suppress allergies. The central nervous system is especially sensitive to antihistamines. Often, these drugs cause profound alterations of mood, not for the better. They make people depressed, grouchy, lethargic, drowsy, and unable to think clearly. Some of them are related chemically to major tranquilizers like Thorazine and produce similar effects on mood. The sedation caused by antihistamines is likely to interfere with driving and other activities requiring concentration, clear thinking, and good reflexes. These effects are intensified by the simultaneous use of alcohol and other depressants. Recently, new antihistamines have appeared that do not enter the brain. The best known of these is terfenadine (Seldane). It does not cause sedation and depression but often causes headaches and other uncomfortable side effects. It is much more expensive than older antihistamines.

Despite their tendency to put people in bad moods, antihistamines are among the most widely consumed of all medical drugs, and neither doctors nor patients think of them as psychoactive. Furthermore, antihistamines are common ingredients of many over-the-counter preparations, such as cold remedies and sleeping aids; they sometimes even arrive in the mail as free samples of these products. Anyone suffering from chronic depression and lethargy should make sure that they are not consuming these chemicals in one form or another. Allergy sufferers should also know that allergic symptoms frequently respond to nondrug treatments, such as changes in diet and mental state, making it possible to avoid antihistamines entirely.

A few drugs in this class are used specifically to prevent motion sickness. Dimenhydrinate (Dramamine) is the best known. Like its relatives, it often makes people drowsy and puts them in unwelcome states of mind.

Oddly enough, one antihistamine is used by some people, mostly junkies, to get high. It is tripelennamine, sold under the brand names PBZ and Pyribenzamine. Because a common form of it is a blue tablet, it is known as "blues" on the street. The combination of morphine and blues is called "blue velvet"; some junkies like to inject it intravenously. A more popular combination is the synthetic opiate pentazocine (Talwin) and PBZ, which is known as "T's and B's" or "T's and blues" and is also taken intravenously. Except for this strange practice, recreational use of antihistamines is rare to nonexistent.

The use of antihistamines in high doses or over long periods seems unwise. These drugs have known toxicity on the physical body, and no one should spend more time than necessary in the mental states that they produce.

Corticosteroids (Cortisone and Relatives)

Besides producing adrenaline, the adrenal glands secrete other hormones that control metabolism and body chemistry. This group of hormones comes from the gland's outer layer, or cortex, so the principal one is called cortisone. Cortisone and its relatives all have a distinctive molecular structure known as the steroid nucleus (which they share with the male and female sex hormones described later in this chapter). Pharmacologists have learned to make many semisynthetic drugs with this same structure, starting with raw materials found in certain plants. As a group, these drugs are all called corticosteroids, or, simply, steroids, both the endogenous ones and the manmade ones.

One of the dramatic effects of corticosteroids is to reduce inflammation and certain allergic reactions, such as skin rashes. Pharmacologists have maximized this action in some of the new steroids that they have created in laboratories. When these drugs are applied topically — that is, when they are put on the skin — they are reasonably safe and sometimes miraculously effective. Doctors also frequently prescribe steroids for systemic use — that is, to be taken internally. There are clear indications for such use, but because steroids seem almost to have magic powers, doctors tend to overprescribe them, sometimes dispensing them for mild cases of poison ivy, diaper rash, back pain, and other conditions not severe enough to warrant their use.

The trouble is that the desirable anti-inflammatory properties of steroids are just one of many actions of these powerful hormones. Even in moderate doses, systemic steroids can drastically upset the chemical balance of the body and cause serious toxicity, including death. They can also shut off the body's production of its own steroids with such consequences as increased susceptibility to stress and infection.

The adverse physical side effects of steroids are well known to doctors, but less attention is paid to their psychoactivity. These drugs can produce extreme euphoria, resembling the manic phase of manic-depressive psychosis. In such cases, judgment can be severely impaired and behavior can become erratic and illogical. With continued use, this initial euphoria may turn into intense depression. Steroids can make some people psychotic or suicidal. Not everyone taking steroids systemically experiences these dramatic reactions, but many probably experience more subtle changes in mood; nervousness, insomnia, depression, and other mental changes are common with long-term use. People with a history of psychiatric problems should be cautious about taking steroids. Everyone should be aware that these compounds are among the strongest drugs known and so should be saved for the treatment of really serious illness.

Anabolic Steroids

Male sex hormones are also called anabolic steroids because they stimulate anabolism, the building-up phase of metabolism. Under their influence, protein synthesis increases in bone, muscle, and skin, leading to increased bone density, muscle mass, and skin tone. These hormones are also androgens — that is, they stimulate the development of male sex characteristics: facial and body hair, male distribution of fat and muscle, deep voice, and so forth. (Female hormones — estrogens and progesterone — are actually derivatives of androgens; both types of hormones are present in both sexes and in delicate balance. Estrogens produce female characteristics but, except for maintaining bone density in women, do not have the general anabolic actions of androgens.)

For some time now, male athletes and body builders have taken anabolic steroids to increase muscle bulk and enhance performance. In fact, the practice has become astonishingly common. Most physicians deplore this use of steroid hormones, but until recently, some wrote prescriptions for them to all comers. In 1991, the Drug Enforcement Administration made anabolic steroids controlled substances, ending legal prescription of them. A black market now supplies both oral and injectable forms of these drugs, but they are of questionable purity. In our experience, peo-

ple determined to use these drugs cannot be dissuaded by warnings about their harmful effects. The promise of rapid development of big muscles and a powerful body image is totally
seductive, especially for teen-agers and young men. Competitive
body builders say that they cannot take the chance of not using steroids since everyone else is using them.

Anabolic steroids may be hazardous to both physical and mental health. They weaken resistance by unbalancing the body's hormonal system and predispose those who take them to weakness
rather than strength in later life. They commonly increase aggression, possibly encouraging violent behavior (" 'roid rage"). They
may also undermine sexual potency and desire. Women athletes
who take steroids may become masculinized; for example, they
may develop deep voices and facial hair.

Proponents of steroids say that adverse effects are rare and that
medical science has failed to document any serious consequences
of use. They say that instead of condemning nonmedical use of
anabolic steroids, researchers should be trying to invent new compounds that are anabolic without being significantly androgenic.

Cough Suppressants

The oldest and most effective drugs for coughs are the opiates.
They directly depress the center in the brain that controls the
cough reflex. It is not always a good idea to stop people from
coughing; sometimes they need to expel material from the respiratory tract. If an unproductive cough continues, however, it
should be stopped.

The most common opiate prescribed for coughs is codeine, a
relatively less powerful one that is reasonably active by mouth.
Because of the danger of dependence, doctors do not prescribe
opiates casually. Pharmacologists have tried to vary the molecules
of opiates to come up with new compounds that will suppress
coughs but not cause euphoria or dependence. Some of their
inventions are available by prescription, such as hydrocodone,
a semisynthetic derivative of codeine. Although these narcotic

> I've had asthma all my life and am allergic to just about
> everything . . . As a child I took a lot of codeine for coughs.
> For the past ten years, I've been on Hycodan, which I un-
> derstand contains a narcotic [hydrocodone]. Originally,
> I took one tablet four times a day; now I take two, four
> times a day. If I try to cut down the dose, I start coughing
> and get really congested. Also, I get upset and can't sleep.
>
> If I think about it, I guess I know I'm addicted, but I
> don't like to face that. I've never had anything to do with
> drugs.
>
> — fifty-two-year-old woman, university guidance counselor

cough suppressants carry warnings about dependence, patients
and doctors may not appreciate the reality of the risk until it is too
late. Also, these drugs, like other narcotics, are depressants and
can interfere with thinking and motor coordination. If they are the
only thing that works for a bad cough, they should be taken intermittently or for only a few days in a row so as to avoid habitual use.

Gastrointestinal Drugs

One of the commonest drugs used to treat intestinal cramps
and diarrhea is Lomotil, a combination of a synthetic opiate called
diphenoxylate and atropine, one of the constituents of nightshade
plants. Both of these drugs reduce the movement of the intestines
by paralyzing the nerves that control them. Diphenoxylate is a
close chemical relative of meperidine (Demerol), one of the strong
medical narcotics. Like its relative, diphenoxylate can cause depression of the nervous system that may be intensified by simultaneous use of other depressants. It can also cause euphoria and dependence. Many patients who take Lomotil for intestinal upset
experience narcotic effects on mood but have no idea that they are
using an opiate.

Atropine by itself has little psychoactivity in low doses; most people find high doses unpleasant. Some combination drugs mix atropine with other nightshade derivatives, including scopolamine, the main psychoactive principle of the nightshade family. Donnatal is an example of such a mixture; it also includes some phenobarbital as a sedative. Doctors frequently maintain patients on these drugs, especially patients with ulcers, gastrointestinal spasms, and urinary disorders. Rarely do doctors or patients consider the potential of these treatments to affect mood and thought, but as noted in the section on deliriants (see pages 157–63), nightshade drugs can influence the mind profoundly. The psychoactive effect most likely to be noticed by people who take these drugs is drowsiness, but over time or in high dosage, they may cause more bizarre changes.

Bronchodilators

Bronchodilators are drugs that open the airways in the respiratory tract. They are widely prescribed as pills and aerosol inhalers to patients with asthma to relieve the wheezing and difficulty in breathing characteristic of that disease. Most of these drugs work by stimulating the sympathetic nervous system, which regulates the muscular walls of the bronchial tubes. As a result, in addition to their desired effect, they commonly cause stimulation, anxiety, jitteriness, and insomnia. Patients often dislike these side effects but have no alternatives to the drugs if they want to breathe.

Another problem with the stimulant bronchodilators is their strong tendency to cause dependence. When the effect of a dose wears off, bronchial constriction increases as a reaction to the drug, making further doses necessary. Asthmatics frequently inhale bronchodilators throughout the day, in addition to taking them regularly by mouth. This frequency of use increases the risks of addiction and mood change.

One of the most widely prescribed of these drugs — theophylline — has recently come under close scrutiny as a possible cause of bizarre and violent behavior. Theophylline is the active principle of tea and is a near relative of caffeine. For many years, most asthmatics have swallowed large daily doses of this stimulant, which was considered a safe and effective drug. Now, with increasing evidence that it can produce serious behavioral changes, its days of use as a medical treatment are numbered.

"Mild" Analgesics

Pharmacologists have been unable to come up with analgesics (pain relievers) of medium strength to fill the gap between aspirin and morphine. They have given us several derivatives of opiates that they claim are more powerful than aspirin but safer and less addicting than morphine. If these drugs are effective at controlling pain, however, they always turn out to be attractive to opiate addicts and are likely to cause dependence.

One such drug is propoxyphene (Darvon), a prescription analgesic widely used in recent years. Sometimes it is combined with aspirin and caffeine to make it more effective. Despite the enthusiastic claims of its manufacturer, most doctors and patients have found Darvon to be not much more effective than aspirin. (Some even feel that when it is combined with aspirin, it is the aspirin that does most of the work.) Besides, the abuse potential of Darvon is of the same sort as that of the strong narcotic analgesics. It took some time for doctors to acknowledge the existence of Darvon abuse, but they are now very familiar with it and much more cautious about dispensing the drug.

In addition to the drugs in these categories, many other prescription drugs may have psychoactive effects, even if doctors, pharmacologists, and manufacturers don't recognize them. Sometimes these effects show up in many patients who take a drug, sometimes in only a few. If you begin a course of prescription drug treatment and experience sleepiness, depression, highs, unusual dreams, or other mental changes that you cannot account for, the drug may be responsible. To prove it, you would have to stop the drug and, after an interval, start it again to see if there is a relationship between it and the symptoms.

Over-the-Counter (OTC) Preparations

Cough Syrups

OTC cough syrups are of varied composition. Some contain no obviously psychoactive drugs. Others contain known depressants, such as alcohol and chloroform; stimulants such as pseudo-ephedrine; antihistamines; and derivatives of opiates considered to be nonnarcotic. Sometimes, people who are desperate for drugs and who cannot get anything better consume overdoses of these preparations in an effort to get high.

The principal OTC cough suppressant is a drug called dextromethorphan, a relative of codeine that quiets the cough center but is not supposed to produce euphoria, dependence, or the other characteristic effects of narcotics. Some people use it to get high, however. It is in Robitussin cough syrup and Coricidin cold tablets ("red devils," "triple-Cs") and can be found on the street in pure form called DXM. Users take large amounts to produce a zombie-like state called "dexing" or "robotripping." The addictive potential and medical harmfulness of excessive use of dextromethorphan are not known.

Cold Remedies

Capsules and tablets for relieving symptoms of colds account for a large percentage of OTC drug sales. Like the cough syrups, cold remedies are a mixed bag of different formulas and strengths. Common ingredients are antihistamines, aspirin and other pain relievers, nightshade drugs to dry up excess secretion in the nose and throat, and caffeine and pseudoephedrine or synephrine to offset the sedative effects of the other ingredients. Usually, these mixtures are packaged in multicolored tablets and flashy capsules to make them look exotic and powerful. Whether they affect the course of a cold or significantly reduce the symptoms is questionable. (Even when they do suppress symptoms, they may actually prolong colds by making people less aware of their illness and less likely to take good care of themselves.) What is more certain is that OTC cold remedies can affect mood, usually in undesirable ways. Alternate methods of treating colds to avoid these problems include taking hot baths, forcing fluids, eating less, increasing rest, and decreasing stress and stimulation.

Nasal Decongestants

One of the physical effects of stimulants is to constrict blood vessels in the nose and sinuses. This constriction shrinks those tissues, allowing freer passage of air. The effect is temporary and, when the stimulant wears off, is usually followed by an opposite reaction, or "rebound," in which the nasal passages become more blocked than before. This pattern is similar to the one that occurs with the bronchodilator drugs described earlier.

Early nasal inhalers contained strips of paper impregnated with amphetamine. Many users experienced general stimulation from them, some got high, and some became dependent. Some even broke open the containers and extracted the amphetamine in order to put it into their bodies in other ways. Eventually, manufacturers stopped using amphetamine in nasal inhalers, replacing it with other drugs supposed to be less stimulating and less addictive.

Today, the OTC inhalers and sprays sold to unblock stuffy noses are not considered psychoactive. Some of the inhalers contain no drugs but only aromatic substances such as menthol. They may be pleasant to use but are not nearly as effective as chemicals that constrict blood vessels. The sprays and those inhalers that do contain drugs certainly work in the short run, but though the manufacturers claim otherwise, they are still stimulants and frequently cause dependence.

Not everyone experiences general stimulation from these products, but those who do may come to use them habitually. Probably, a greater risk of dependence arises from the temporary nature of the relief that they offer. If people continue to use them to treat the rebound that follows the initial dose, they quickly find themselves unable to breathe without them. Longer-acting preparations may be safer in this respect.

A few oral forms of decongestants are available, for example, pseudoephedrine (Sudafed), a close relative of the natural stimulant ephedrine. Since it goes into the mouth rather than the nose, it is less likely to cause rebound and dependence, but for some people and in high doses, it is definitely a stimulant. Synephrine, a product of the bitter orange tree, is also a stimulant.

Appetite Suppressants

We mentioned these oral forms of stimulants at the end of Chapter 6. Until recently, they contained ephedrine, sometimes combined with caffeine, and are packaged and named to look like amphetamines.

OTC Uppers

Pure caffeine is sold in most drugstores — for much more than it is worth — in clever disguises meant to suggest powerful amphetamines. For example, a product called Caffedrine, in large green-and-white time-release capsules, looks just like pharmaceutical Dexamyl. No doubt, some people who buy it resell it on the black market as Dexamyl to gullible buyers. Older and more straightforward products are Vivarin and No-Doz, in the form of simple white tablets. If these products are more effective than coffee or tea, it is only because people believe in pills.

OTC Downers

A variety of products is available in drugstores to promote sleep at night (Nytol, Sominex, Unisom). They are widely used as nonprescription analogs of the stronger minor tranquilizers and sleeping pills. All of them contain antihistamines, usually diphenhydramine (Benadryl), pyrilamine, or doxylamine. As we have pointed out, these chemicals are not innocuous and tend to affect mental function in unpleasant ways. They will make people drowsy but can produce depression as well and can be habit-forming.

We favor less toxic remedies for insomnia, such as increased exercise during the day, decreased use of stimulants, especially in the evening (remember to read the labels of any pain pills, cold tablets, and other remedies to see if they contain caffeine or other stimulants), relaxation techniques, warm baths, and simple nutritional supplements such as calcium and magnesium tablets, which relax many people when taken at bedtime.

Analgesics

Although nonnarcotic pain relievers do not directly affect the mind, they can change moods dramatically by decreasing discomfort and so can be habit-forming. The common OTC analgesics, such as aspirin and acetaminophen (Tylenol), are effective remedies for occasional use, but when pain persists, people should seek to identify and treat the causes rather than rely on these drugs. Some analgesic compounds contain caffeine solely for its stimulant and mood-elevating effects.

OTC drugs are big business and are not regulated in the same way as prescription drugs. Manufacturers can get them on the market without doing much to prove their effectiveness, can deemphasize their adverse effects, and can make outrageous claims in their advertising. Most people assume that the products heaped on drugstore counters are mild but effective, nontoxic, and nonaddictive. Those are not safe assumptions. Anyone who uses OTC drugs should know what they contain and how they affect the body and mind.

Herbal Remedies

With increasing interest in alternatives to regular medicine, the marketing of herbal remedies and medicinal plants has boomed.

Most health food stores have herb departments, and some of the products they sell are even appearing in drugstores and supermarkets. Many are just pleasant herbal teas, such as peppermint and chamomile, without significant drug effects, but a few are really psychoactive. In Chapter 6, we discussed *guaraná*, maté, yohimbe, and ephedra, all stimulants.

A plant with the opposite effect is valerian; its root is a strong natural sedative that does not depress vital functions or cause the kind of dependence that sleeping pills do. Preparations of valerian root, including tinctures and capsules, are obtainable at health food stores. Valerian has a strange, musty odor that some people find disagreeable, but it is easy to take as a capsule or tincture and does work. For people who need nighttime sedatives, it is probably a better choice than more dangerous synthetic drugs.

Kava, or kava-kava, is another herbal depressant whose effect is of a more general anesthetic nature than a sedative. It is the root of a large tropical plant related to black pepper and cultivated on many islands of the South Pacific. Natives there make drinks from fresh or dried kava root and consume them as ritual and social drugs. Preparations of the fresh root are more powerful, putting users into a pleasant, dreamy state while numbing their bodies. Drinks made from the dried root are more relaxing than intoxicating. Kava ceremonies take place at night and often bring large groups of people together for the main social event of island life. Only dried kava is available outside the South Pacific. Herb stores sell it as a coarse powder or larger chips of root. When chewed, dried kava makes the mouth numb and may be relaxing. Some people brew it into a tea, which they like as a mild downer.

In the 1990s, many extracts of kava appeared on the market in capsule form. In Germany, both prescription and over-the-counter versions were in wide use as natural antianxiety agents. Then reports began to accumulate of cases of severe liver disease in people using kava; as a result, its popularity has dropped off sharply. We do not know the exact cause of these reactions, which mainly occurred in Europe. Perhaps the alcohol extracts of kava in use there contain toxic compounds not present in water extracts. Until the issue is settled, people with a history of liver problems should avoid kava.

One of the most famous of the plant drugs is ginseng, obtained from the roots of several species of woodland plants, one from China and Korea and another from the northeastern United States. People in Asia have used ginseng for centuries, paying high prices for the best quality roots and valuing them as a general tonic. They believe that ginseng increases vitality, resistance to disease, and longevity. It is especially used by men, and those who use it often say it increases sexual power, particularly as they grow older.

Ginseng has only recently become popular in the West, and Western scientists still do not understand it very well. They are convinced that ginseng has effects, but they don't yet know what all of them are. One source of confusion is that commercial products vary tremendously in potency; some have no activity at all. For some people, ginseng is a strong stimulant. It may raise blood pressure and should be used with caution by people with high blood pressure. Other users claim that it tones their muscles and skin and increases their physical endurance. "Siberian ginseng" is not true ginseng but comes from a related plant; it is less of a stimulant.

The effects of ginseng are cumulative, often not becoming apparent unless the drug is used regularly for weeks or months. The chemistry of the root is very complex. Some compounds in it may affect the production of steroid hormones, which could explain the results that users report. In any case, ginseng is a drug, not just a dietary supplement or new-age hoax, even though it now appears in everything from toothpaste to soda. If you want to try ginseng, avoid these senseless preparations and be prepared to spend a lot of money for whole roots, capsules, or extracts of reliable potency.

Smart Drugs

Since many people in our society turn to drugs for solutions to everything from heartburn to boredom, it is not surprising that they would get excited about drugs that are supposed to boost intelligence, memory, and concentration. Students are always looking for ways to increase their brain power. Users of alcohol, pot, and cocaine worry about the adverse effects of those substances on their minds. Some people approaching middle age become obsessed with extending their lives, enhancing their declining sexuality, and fortifying their brains against the ravages of old age. For all of these concerns, there is a new answer: smart drugs.

Smart drugs are a diverse group of compounds. Some are prescription drugs marketed openly in this country. Others are prescription drugs from other countries and are not generally available here but can be obtained by mail order or from Mexico. Still others can be had in health food stores and from other sources selling nutritional supplements.

Two kinds of smart drugs are nootropics and cognitive enhancers. The word *nootropic* (meaning "mind-turning") was coined to describe substances believed to improve learning and memory without affecting the brain in other ways and without causing toxicity, even at high doses. "Cognitive enhancer" is a vaguer term for substances that might improve general mental functioning.

Many of the smart drugs have been around for years, but information on them became widely available only in the 1990s. The media first began paying attention to them at this time, probably because of the appearance of "smart bars" in San Francisco and other cities. Smart bars are clubs that serve nonalcoholic drinks spiked with smart drugs. Who goes to smart bars? Students studying for exams are frequent patrons, but all sorts of people wander in to try the concoctions.

Here is a selection of some of the more popular smart drugs.

Piracetam and Relatives (Oxiracetam, Aniracetam, Pramiracetam, and Pyroglutamate)

These drugs, known collectively as pyrrolidone derivatives, are the most important family of nootropics. Smart-drug enthusiasts say they cause remarkable enhancement of memory. No one knows

> Piracetam keeps me alert when I am driving. It also helps
> me formulate new and different ideas when I am taking
> essay tests in school.
>
> — twenty-one-year-old woman, student

how they work, but they may affect nerve pathways in the brain
that use acetylcholine as a neurotransmitter. Acetylcholine declines
with age and may account for slowed mental function in the el-
derly. Users say piracetam is a central nervous system stimulant that
wakes up the brain. They claim that it has no toxicity or addictive
properties. Piracetam is not sold in the United States but can
be ordered by mail or purchased over the counter at Mexican
pharmacies.

DHEA (Dehydroepiandrosterone)

DHEA is an endogenous steroid hormone made in the adrenal
glands. It is related to male sex hormones and has weak androgenic activity. Smart-drug enthusiasts say that it combats obesity,
aging, and cancer, extends life, and keeps you looking youthful.
They also think that it can protect brain cells from the degenerative changes of old age. Research to back up these claims is lacking. The drug is available from "buying clubs" that supply unapproved drugs to AIDS patients. (DHEA is also supposed to boost
immunity.)

DMAE (Dimethylaminoethanol)

This endogenous substance, present in small amounts in the
brain, also occurs in some fish (anchovies and sardines). It is described as a nutrient that has mild stimulant properties and can
also elevate mood, increase intelligence, and counteract fatigue.
Like piracetam, it may work on acetylcholine pathways in the
brain. Health food stores sell DMAE as a nutritional supplement.

Hydergine

Hydergine is a pharmaceutical drug, derived from ergot, and is available by prescription in the United States as a cognitive enhancer for people suffering from mental impairment as a result of age or brain injury. It has little toxicity, and its mechanism of action is unknown. Although many doctors question its efficacy, the drug has a large following among smart-drug fans, who believe that it improves memory and learning and protects the brain from weakening with age. Hydergine is quite expensive.

Selegiline (Eldepryl, Deprenyl)

A newer prescription drug, recently introduced for the treatment of Parkinson's disease, Eldepryl has gained a strong reputation as another smart drug, one that wakes up the brain, increasing alertness and energy and enhancing all mental functions. Eldepryl is metabolized to amphetamine and methamphetamine in the body, which probably accounts for these effects.

Vasopressin (Diapid)

Vasopressin is an endogenous hormone produced by the pituitary gland. Also known as antidiuretic hormone, or ADH, it causes the body to retain urine. Doctors prescribe it in the form of a nasal spray to treat patients with a rare disease called diabetes insipidus, marked by frequent urination. Smart-drug enthusiasts say that vasopressin spray also affects the mind, improving attention, concentration, and memory. In addition, they say, it instantly counteracts the crash that follows the use of stimulant drugs and the grogginess caused by high doses of marijuana and alcohol. Vasopressin nasal spray can give you a number of uncomfortable side effects, including nasal irritation, runny nose, headache, and abdominal cramps.

It is difficult to assess the benefits and risks of smart drugs, because not enough research exists on them. Although doctors question their safety, especially when used in the combinations that their fans prefer, safety may be less of a concern than efficacy. It is not at all clear that these substances really have the beneficial effects claimed by their promoters, and we do not have enough information to know just what are the effects of long-term use.

SUGGESTED READING

Two useful books on medical drugs are *The Essential Guide to Prescription Drugs* by James W. Long (sixth edition; New York: Harper-Collins, 2002) and *Over Dose: The Case Against the Drug Companies: Prescription Drugs, Side Effects, and Your Health* by Jay S. Cohen (New York: Penguin USA, 2001).

Is There No Place on Earth for Me? by Susan Sheehan (Boston: Houghton Mifflin, 1982) is a vivid case history of a young schizophrenic woman who, during repeated hospitalizations, is treated with ever-increasing doses of virtually all the major tranquilizers then in use.

Prozac Backlash: Overcoming the Dangers of Prozac, Zoloft, Paxil, and Other Antidepressants with Safe, Effective Alternatives by Joseph Glenmullen (New York: Simon & Schuster, 2000) is a provocative look at the treatment of depression. Lauren Slater's *Prozac Diary* (London: Penguin, 1999) is an excellent personal account of Prozac use. So is Elizabeth Wurtzel's *Prozac Nation: Young and Depressed in America: A Memoir* (New York: Riverhead Books, 1997). Finally, see *Listening to Prozac: A Psychiatrist Explores Antidepressant Drugs and the Remaking of the Self* by Peter D. Kramer, M.D. (New York: Viking Penguin, 1993).

Also, see *Pills a Go Go: Fiendish Investigation into Pill Marketing, Art, History, and Consumption* by Jim Hogshire (Venice, Calif.: Feral House, 1999) for an informative account of pharmaceutical drugs.

An excellent all-around guide to herbal medicine is *The New Age Herbalist: How to Use Herbs for Healing, Nutrition, Body Care, and Relaxation* by Richard Mabey and Michael McIntyre (New York: Fireside, 1988). See also the periodical *HerbalGram* from the American Botanical Council (www.herbalgram.org)(last accessed February 2004).

The best references on smart drugs are *Smart Drugs & Nutrients* by

Ward Dean, M.D., and John Morgenthaler (Petaluma, Calif.: Smart Publications, 1991), and *Smart Drugs II: The Next Generation: New Drugs and Nutrients to Improve Your Memory and Increase Your Intelligence* by Ward Dean, M.D., John Morgenthaler, and Steven William Fowkes (Petaluma, Calif.: Smart Publications, 1993).

12. Problems with Drugs

I N THE PRECEDING CHAPTERS we have discussed the risks and problems associated with using specific drugs. Here we will comment on some more general problems that drug users are apt to encounter.

Uncertainty of Dose and Quality

When drugs come from legal sources, they are likely to be pure, of standard dosage, and correctly labeled. Yet even medical drugs can be outdated and mislabeled, and they sometimes contain fillers and colorings that can be harmful to some people. These problems are insignificant compared with those of black-market drugs, which are regularly cut with impurities, are of uncertain dosage, and are often completely misrepresented to the buyer.

Buying pills and powders on the street is a risky business at best. Not only do you have to deal with unsavory characters and participate in illegal transactions, you have no assurance of getting what you pay for. If you are lucky, what you buy will contain some of what it's supposed to contain and be cut with nothing more dangerous than starch or sugar. If you are less lucky, the pills and powders will be inactive, and if you aren't lucky at all, they will contain something actively harmful. Not only are you likely to get ripped off on the black market, you can also wind up in a hospital emergency room. People who inject street drugs are in greatest danger, because putting impurities directly into the bloodstream gives the body no chance to deal with them.

Some help with these uncertainties is offered by private testing labs that will analyze samples of drugs for a reasonable fee while protecting the customer's anonymity. Drug enforcement authorities will not allow these labs to give quantitative results, however, so that although you may find out what is in your material, you still won't know how potent it is. About the only way to be sure that you are getting what you want in the way of nonmedical drugs is to grow your own drug plants or collect them in the wild. Otherwise, you must know your sources; remember that the black market encourages deception and misrepresentation, and be extremely cautious about consuming any substance obtained on the street.

Mixing Drugs

In a few instances, the results of mixing psychoactive drugs are clear. For example, we have noted the additive effects of combining alcohol and downers or tranquilizers. In many more cases, the effects of drug combinations are unpredictable, depending more on the individual and on set and setting than on pharmacology. Mixing drugs can increase the problems associated with individual drugs and may create some new ones.

At the very least, drug combinations take getting used to. Many marijuana smokers use alcohol while smoking, but there is no predictable result of this combination. Some people find themselves more stoned, others less stoned, others sleepy or headachy. Until you know the effects of a given combination on *you*, you should proceed cautiously. People who get into bad relationships with drugs often use many drugs together, and some combinations may promote dependency and abuse. People who ingest alcohol and cocaine together often wind up taking more of both than they would if they used either by itself. Coffee and cigarettes together form a very stubborn habit — it is almost as if one triggers a desire for the other.

These days it is not unusual to see groups of people drinking alcohol, snorting coke, and smoking pot, as well as using tobacco, drinking coffee, and eating chocolate — all at the same time and in large doses. Such polydrug consumption tends to promote immoderation and lack of awareness about the nature of the substances being consumed.

Drug combining is a problem in medicine as well. Medical patients often receive many prescription drugs simultaneously, and doctors are often ignorant about how they interact. Interactions of medical drugs and recreational drugs are also largely unknown. If you are taking medical drugs, keep in mind that they might change your reaction to recreational drugs. If you use recreational drugs, consider that they might combine unfavorably with prescribed medication.

Medical Problems

Acute Problems

Overdosing and allergic reactions are the most important acute medical problems that can arise from taking psychoactive drugs. Mild overdoses of drugs may produce nausea and vomiting, which usually require no treatment but can be very unpleasant. Large overdoses can cause convulsions, coma, and death; they are medical emergencies requiring immediate treatment in a hospital. Anyone who suddenly loses consciousness or stops breathing after taking a drug should be seen immediately by a doctor. If you are around someone who develops an overdose (OD) reaction, put all legal considerations aside and summon medical help. Never administer more drugs — of *any* type — to a person suffering from overdose.

Intravenous users of drugs are in the greatest danger of dramatic overdose reactions, but people who smoke or snort stimulants and depressants can have them, too, as can people who take very large doses by mouth. Remember that ODs can quickly result in death if hospital treatment is not obtained immediately.

Allergic reactions to drugs take many forms, ranging from itching and swelling of parts of the body to death from asphyxiation because of the swelling of tissues in the windpipe. Serious allergic reactions are very unpredictable and may occur because of contaminants in street drugs as well as the drugs themselves. They may also develop suddenly in people with no prior history of allergy. The symptoms of serious allergic shock are itching in the throat and difficulty in breathing. Again, this is a medical emergency requiring prompt treatment. Anyone who develops such a reaction should be taken to a hospital at once.

Chronic Medical Problems

Any drug used in excess over time can produce illness. Different drugs irritate different systems of the body. In some cases, the association between a drug and a disease is very clear, as it is with alcohol and cirrhosis of the liver or tobacco in the form of cigarettes and lung cancer. We have reviewed these specific physical consequences in previous chapters.

People who use any drug intravenously expose themselves to other risks that are consequences of that method of administration. Putting a crude and unsterilized needle into a vein carries the grave danger of introducing serious infection. Viral hepatitis is probably the most common disease transmitted in this way; it can make people sick for months and cause permanent liver damage. Of even greater concern is AIDS, a fatal, incurable viral infection that destroys the immune system. Intravenous drug users are at risk for this devastating disease if they share needles. A needle used by an infected person can easily transmit the virus to the bloodstream of the next user. Another potential calamity is bacterial endocarditis — an infection of the heart valves. In addition, needle users frequently suffer from abscesses and inflamed and damaged veins. Intramuscular and subcutaneous injections are less dangerous but not without risk. They transmit hepatitis and AIDS equally well.

Smoking anything irritates the throat, bronchial tubes, and lungs. In susceptible individuals, regular smoking of any drug, whether it's tobacco, marijuana, or crack cocaine, can result in respiratory infection, decreased breathing capacity, coughing, bronchitis, and, probably, a greater risk of emphysema and lung cancer. It is also important to keep in mind that smoking puts drugs into the bloodstream and brain very directly, even faster than intravenous injection, making the drugs more toxic and more addicting. Snorting drugs is less direct than intravenous injection but not nearly as safe as oral use; snorting can lead to chronic irritation and erosion of the nasal membranes. Even taken by mouth, some drugs in excess are very irritating. Heavy drinking can cause chronic inflammation of the esophagus and stomach, and too much coffee often gives rise to chronic indigestion.

Heavy users of drugs often have an erratic lifestyle that interferes with regular sleep, good nutrition, and healthful habits of hygiene and exercise. In addition, the drugs they take may suppress appetite, rob the body of vitamins, and upset normal metabolism. All of these effects can lead to such chronic problems as malnutrition, anemia, and decreased resistance to infection. For example, dietary deficiencies in the alcoholic greatly increase the liver's susceptibility to the toxicity of alcohol and contribute to the development of cirrhosis.

Drugs and Pregnancy

Women expose their unborn babies to harm by consuming drugs — any drugs — during pregnancy. Many doctors now advise that expectant women take no drugs whatever during the first three months of pregnancy and as few as possible thereafter. Psychoactive drugs are no exception. In the 1960s, thousands of badly deformed babies were born to women who took the sedative thalidomide, prescribed as a "safe" relaxant and promoter of sleep.

Recreational drugs can also be risky to the fetus, but in most cases, the exact dangers are unknown. It is known that pregnant women who smoke cigarettes have more miscarriages and regularly give birth to babies that weigh less than normal, are more susceptible to respiratory infection, and die more frequently in infancy. Drinking alcohol during pregnancy also increases the rate of birth defects; unfortunately, no one can say what a safe intake of alcohol is for a pregnant woman.

Most of the drugs discussed in this book enter the system of the fetus and affect it in some way. For example, pregnant heroin addicts give birth to addicted babies who must be weaned off opiates in the first few days of life. Given these facts, pregnant women should make an effort to discontinue the use of all psychoactive substances until after they deliver. Even then, they should be careful if they breast-feed, because if they take drugs, their milk may contain amounts high enough to affect a baby. Smoking around an infant can also put drugs into its system, and babies are very sensitive to smoke of all sorts.

Psychiatric Problems

The most common acute psychiatric problem is panic. Typically, people will take a drug, feel it begin to work, and become convinced that they are dying or losing their mind. Panic reactions occur most frequently in people with little drug experience, especially in settings that encourage anxiety. A teen-ager who has never smoked marijuana and is pressured into trying it at a party with strangers is a good candidate for a panic reaction. People who are unaware that someone has slipped them a drug, or who wind up taking much larger doses than they are used to, are also likely to panic. Panic can be very dramatic, making people agitated, helpless, incoherent, and a source of great anxiety to others. People in panic often use the anxiety that they produce in others to fuel their own reactions.

Doctors have sometimes misdiagnosed a panic reaction as an episode of psychosis and have prolonged the episode by confirming the patient's fears of going crazy. People who are panicked need to be reassured and calmed down, preferably by someone with experience, such as a worker at a drug crisis center. Panicky people should not be given sedatives, tranquilizers, or other psychoactive drugs. A hospital emergency room may not be the best place to take people in panic, because it can produce more anxiety than reassurance. Most panic reactions will end quickly, provided that they are recognized for what they are and not intensified by improper management.

Paranoia and "bad trips" are similar to panic reactions and are also mostly products of set and setting. They, too, will subside by themselves if left to run their course.

True psychotic reactions are occasionally triggered by a drug experience, but they are not nearly so common as panic reactions. Just as a first sexual experience or going away from home to college or losing a job can trigger psychosis, so can a stressful drug experience. A person who becomes mentally disturbed after taking a drug and who continues to be disturbed after the effects of the drug wear off should be seen by a professional.

Coming down from drugs ("crashing") presents special problems. People who rely on drugs to feel good may become depressed when the drug wears off. Not only can this depression encourage frequent and abusive drug-taking, but it can also become a chronic psychological problem. Psychiatrists these days often see severely depressed patients who are heavy users of cocaine, and similar depression can occur with the regular use of any psychoactive drug. Depression is often a component of dependence on alcohol and downers, as well as dependence on stimulants.

Crusaders against drugs like to cite many other chronic psychological problems that are supposed to be drug connected, but there is little evidence to support most of their claims. There does seem to be a pharmacological basis for the paranoia and hallucinations that occur in people who shoot amphetamines, and alcohol certainly can cause brain damage, producing distinctive losses of mental function. Heavy use of cocaine and speed often causes personality changes in the direction of irritability, paranoia, and hostility. Major psychological problems may also go hand in hand with heavy consumption of other drugs, but whether they are a direct effect of the drugs is seldom clear.

As an example, there has been much talk of "burn-outs" — young people who are supposed to be casualties of intense use of marijuana, psychedelics, and other illegal drugs. Certainly, there are people who wind up as aimless, confused misfits after using a lot of drugs, but what were these people like before, and what other factors played a role in the change? Many of them were runaways, engaged in unusual sexual experimentation, or joined religious cults in addition to taking drugs. It is easy to blame the drugs, but evidence for their causative role is lacking.

An even better example of the false linking of a problem with a drug is amotivational syndrome. As we have said, it makes much more sense to view heavy marijuana smoking as an expression of amotivation rather than the cause of it. Many amotivated people smoke a lot of marijuana, but so do many well-motivated people. Amotivated people would probably behave in other unproductive ways if marijuana were to disappear. The tendency to see disliked drugs as causes of disapproved behavior is understandable, but it is not valid scientifically and does not help solve the real problems associated with drugs.

Social and Behavioral Problems

Drug-taking can lead to a variety of problems with other people. Many drug users feel guilty about their habits, and their guilt is often an obstacle to intimacy. Using illegal drugs automatically puts people into conflict with social authorities and with parents, teachers, and employers. One of the commonest sources of family tension today is the suspicion or discovery by parents that a child is using drugs. This issue is so emotional that most people are unable to deal with it openly. Often, it creates a climate of distrust and misunderstanding that pervades every aspect of the family's life. Drug use may also isolate children from the mainstream of their peers, driving them into the company of other drug users and limiting their possibilities for balanced social interaction. Of course, children are not the only ones who encounter social prob-

I guess my drug of choice is wine. Two glasses of good
wine put me in just the right state after a trying day. John
drinks wine, too, but for getting high he prefers marijuana.

In the past few years, our different preferences in drugs
have become a problem for us. My not liking marijuana
separates me from John's closest friends and weakens
our relationship. I don't think married people have to do
everything together, but this is something important,
and my inability to share John's highs bothers me. Also,
I find I resent his smoking friends, since I'm the outsider,
the "straight wife," when they are around. Yet I know
that if I object, I will just drive him out of the house to
get high with them elsewhere.

— thirty-five-year-old woman

lems as a result of drug use. Different preferences in recreational
drugs are frequently a source of conflict in couples and can even
result in the breakup of a marriage.

People who abuse drugs, whether legal or illegal, usually find
themselves in social trouble on all levels. The alcoholic father
who can't provide for his family and antagonizes his friends
and coworkers is a classic example. The heroin addict who steals
from a friend to buy his next fix is another. In fact, it is rare to
find a drug abuser who does not provoke some degree of social
conflict.

The drug laws in our society compound the social problems of
people who choose to use illegal drugs. For one, illegal drugs are
very expensive; buying them regularly can significantly drain a
person's economic resources. Second, although casual users of illegal drugs generally obtain their supplies from friends, at some
point the lines of supply connect to the criminal underworld.
Heavy users are apt to be drawn into this sphere, especially if they
begin to sell illicit substances to support their own drug habit.

The dangers of associating with professional drug dealers cannot be overstated. Many dealers handle large sums of cash, are heavily armed, and live in a paranoid world of rip-offs, busts, and informers. Those who grow or smuggle drugs on a large scale are also likely to be caught up in raids by police or federal agents. The ugliness of drug dealing is a direct consequence of laws that criminalize the possession and sale of disapproved substances. Narcotics agents who enforce these laws sometimes behave as disreputably as the people they try to catch, violating civil liberties and recklessly employing violence to chase down "drug traffickers."

Unfortunately, major traffickers are seldom touched by the law, because they are usually rich enough, smart enough, and powerful enough to stay in business. Instead, drug-law enforcement falls disproportionately on small-scale dealers and users. In recent years, so much enforcement has been directed at these people that our court and prison systems are now overwhelmed.

Quite another sort of problem arises from associating with people who are intoxicated on drugs, whether legal or illegal. Intoxication increases the likelihood of accidents and trouble of all kinds. If you keep company and go out in public with drugged friends, you may suffer for their blunders.

Drunk drivers are as dangerous to their passengers and other people on the road as they are to themselves. You have a choice whether to accept rides with them, as you do with drivers who are stoned on pot, tripping on psychedelics, or under the influence of any other drug that might compromise their driving skills. It can be very difficult to refuse a ride with friends because you feel that they are intoxicated, but learning to exercise that choice may save you from injury or death. In Sweden, where alcoholism is common and driving-while-intoxicated laws are strictly enforced, social custom dictates that one member of a group attending a party abstain from drinking in order to be the driver for the evening. The "designated driver" is still a new custom in our society, so individuals who associate with drug users must learn to judge when

> Money is the main reason why my friends and I deal drugs.
> Also, there's a lot of status in it. I mean, if you've got
> money and drugs, you've automatically got power and
> prestige. People say you're crazy to take the risk, but at the
> same time they're envious of you, and that's the truth.
>
> — seventeen-year-old man

they should go their separate ways. By the way, police now have an effective field test to identify drugged drivers. Called the Horizontal Gaze Nystagmus Test, it uses eye movements to detect intoxication by most psychoactive drugs.

These days, because of the widely accepted practice of urine testing, and the newer method of hair sample analysis, recreational users of illegal drugs run a greater risk of exposure than ever before. Many employers require their workers to submit to random urine testing and also screen job applicants in this way. Positive test results commonly mean that you will be fired.

Developmental Problems

The use of drugs by younger and younger children is very alarming to grown-ups. In the 1960s, college students were the main consumers of marijuana; today, pot is commonplace in high schools and, in some parts of the country, even in grade schools. Significant numbers of adolescents have now tried cocaine, alcohol, tobacco, tranquilizers, solvents, psychedelics, and probably more. Drugs have become prevalent in rural as well as urban schools and seem to cut across all class and ethnic boundaries.

Parents, teachers, doctors, and lawmakers generally assume that drug use by the young is especially dangerous. They fear that it will cause permanent physical and psychological damage as well as create whole generations of addicts, criminals, and zombies. It may well be that young people are more susceptible to the adverse effects of psychoactive drugs, but there is little hard evidence on this point. Among Native American groups who use drugs ritually, children are often introduced to natural psychedelics at a very young age without suffering any apparent harm. However, the social context of psychedelic use among these peoples is different from anything that exists in mainstream society.

Psychologists say that adolescence is, at best, a difficult time. Teen-agers must grapple with a host of problems and pressures, some caused by internal hormonal changes, others by the changing expectations of society as they approach maturity. One concern of psychologists is that the addition of drugs to this already turbulent process will make it significantly harder. Another concern is that young people will use drugs to avoid facing the conflicts that must be resolved if they are to develop into healthy adults. At the moment, there are no studies of adults who began using marijuana and other drugs while they were kids. Perhaps when such studies are done, the results will allay some of the worst fears. However, until then, it is no doubt safer to assume that children and adolescents *are* at greater risk and that, below a certain age, drug-taking may impair normal mental and emotional development. At the very least, using psychoactive drugs in childhood and adolescence to avoid boredom, conflict, and other bad feelings is likely to establish unhealthy patterns of drug-taking that will persist and cause problems in later life.

Legal Problems

Getting arrested for possession of drugs can be devastating. At best, it can absorb a great deal of time and money (including sei-

> I have been a criminal ever since the day I smoked my first joint.
>
> — forty-year-old man, landscape architect

> To think that a man should be allowed a gun and not a drug!
>
> — **Alexander Trocchi, from his novel *Cain's Book* (1960)**

zure of your house, car, and other assets); at worst, it can subject you to the horrors of prison and leave a permanent blot on your record. Current drug laws are the product of society's fears and prejudices and would certainly strike an unbiased observer as irrational, if not insane. In some states, people convicted for small-scale dealing of drugs such as cocaine and LSD are treated more harshly by the law than rapists, armed robbers, and even murderers. We think that the drug laws have done much more harm than good, but the fact is that they exist and are enforced. The current war on drugs has spawned tougher drug laws, with mandatory minimum sentences and "zero tolerance" of even casual users' possessing small amounts of marijuana. People who share drugs with friends may be considered dealers by the law, subject to heavy penalties if convicted.

If you run afoul of the drug laws, waste no time in getting the advice and help of a lawyer who specializes in this area. If you have no idea where to turn for information and have little or no money, contact a local office of the Legal Aid Society, which is listed in the telephone directory of most cities. Legal Aid can advise you and help you find a lawyer. The National Organization to Reform Marijuana Laws (NORML) is a good source for legal information and assistance. You can contact the group at www.norml.org/index.cfm (last accessed April 2004).

Dependency and Addiction

A chief characteristic of a bad relationship with a drug is difficulty in leaving it alone. Dependence on drugs is common and provokes so much censure and fear that it makes it hard to see that

Nothing is more destructive of respect for the government
and the law of the land than passing laws which cannot
be enforced.

— Albert Einstein

dependence is a basic human problem not limited to drugs. People can become dependent on many substances and practices; sources of pleasure are obviously the most frequent: food, sex, drugs. People can also become dependent on certain experiences, such as falling in love or having sex, seeking them out compulsively to the exclusion of other activities. It is also easy for people to become dependent on other people. Such personal relationships share many features of drug dependence, including tolerance (diminished pleasure with frequent exposure) and withdrawal (difficulty separating). People become dependent on jogging, gambling, watching television, shopping, working, and talking on the telephone. These observations suggest that dependence has more to do with human beings than with drugs. When people talk about the "addictive potential" of a substance, what they are really talking about is the tendency of human beings to get addicted to it.

The terms *addiction* and *dependence* are used loosely today. Properly speaking, drug addiction is a special kind of dependence, marked by physical changes: tolerance that requires increasing doses of the drug to achieve the same effect and a withdrawal syndrome if the drug is discontinued. People who become dependent on marijuana do not show tolerance and withdrawal as heroin addicts do. This fact has led many experts to talk about "psychological dependence." However, psychological dependence is a fuzzy concept. How does it differ from doing something repeatedly because you like it? Is there anything wrong with doing something you like repeatedly if it does not hurt you?

The real problem with dependence is that it limits personal freedom.

Of course, everyone is dependent on food, water, and other people; no one can ever be completely self-sufficient. Dependencies become a problem when they take up vast amounts of time, money, and energy; create guilt and anxiety; and control one's life. It is easy for people to ignore the extent to which dependencies control their lives; sometimes other people can see the problem more clearly.

Dependence on anything is not easy to break. More often than not, people simply switch dependencies, substituting one for another without achieving greater freedom. Still, it is no doubt better to be dependent on exercising, say, than on watching TV. Perhaps the tendency to become dependent is incurable, but to a certain extent people can choose what they are dependent on. Tobacco addicts who give up smoking by becoming compulsive joggers may not be any freer, but they may live longer, be healthier, and feel better about themselves.

Dependence on drugs may be better than dependence on some things and worse than dependence on others, but such value judgments are difficult to make without reference to particular individuals and situations. Is it better to be dependent on skydiving or snorting coke? On masturbating or eating chocolate? On fighting or shooting heroin?

Good relationships with drugs do not involve dependence. Once you become dependent on a drug, it may be difficult or impossible to get back into a good relationship with it. Most experts on alcoholism say that alcoholics cannot learn to be social drinkers; their only choice is between continued alcoholism and abstinence. Most people who smoke cigarettes nonaddictively never were addicted smokers; they formed a good relationship with cigarettes and maintained it. The surest way to avoid dependence on drugs is never to use them. If you do use drugs and want to avoid becoming dependent, you will have to take steps to create a good relationship with them right from the start.

The treatment of drug addiction has become big business. Private treatment centers charge thousands of dollars a week to get people off cocaine, alcohol, marijuana, narcotics, and tranquilizers. Twelve-step programs modeled on Alcoholics Anonymous have proliferated in all cities, and special programs now exist to treat the relatives of dependent persons — Adult Children of Alcoholics and Codependents Anonymous, for example. Despite the boom in the treatment industry, the rate of addiction has only increased.

We think that addiction is a basic human problem whose roots go very deep. Most of us have at some point been wounded, no matter what kind of family we grew up in or what kind of society we live in. We long for a sense of completeness and wholeness and most often search for satisfaction outside of ourselves. Ironically, whatever satisfaction we gain from drugs, food, sex, money, and other "sources" of pleasure really comes from inside of us. That is, we project our power onto external substances and activities, allowing them to make us feel better temporarily. This is a very strange sort of magic. We give away our power in exchange for a transient sense of wholeness, then suffer because the object of our craving seems to control us. Addiction can be cured only when we consciously experience this process, reclaim our power, and recognize that our wounds must be healed from within.

SUGGESTED READING

The autobiographical books listed in the Suggested Reading sections of preceding chapters give firsthand descriptions of problems with various drugs.

Two books written about teen-agers and drugs are *Smoking, Drinking, and Drug Use in Young Adulthood: The Impact of New Freedoms and New Responsibilities* by Jerald G. Bachman et al. (Mahwah, N.J.: L. Erlbaum Associates, 1997) and *Dirty: A Search for Answers Inside America's Teenage Drug Epidemic* by Meredith Maran (San Francisco: Harper, 2003). For a fictional account of drug dependence among high-school students, see *Go Ask Alice* by Anonymous (New York: Avon, 1972).

The National Center on Addiction and Substance Abuse at Columbia University (CASA) has published the excellent 2003 report "Teen Cigarette Smoking and Marijuana Use." This and other reports may be downloaded for free from www.casacolumbia.org (last accessed February 2004).

The National Institute on Drug Abuse, in conjunction with the University of Michigan's Institute for Social Research, has published a comprehensive two-part report monitoring drug use from 1975 to 2002, *Monitoring the Future* (Rockville, Md.: National Institute on Drug Abuse, National Institutes of Health, 2003). The first volume examines drug use among secondary school students, and the second looks at people aged nineteen to forty. Both may be downloaded at no charge from http://monitoringthefuture.org/pubs/monographs/vol1_2002.pdf and http://monitoringthefuture.org/pubs/monographs/vol2_2002.pdf (last accessed April 22, 2004).

Coming Clean: Overcoming Addiction Without Treatment by Robert Granfield and William Cloud (New York: New York University Press, 1999) is an important account of forty-six individuals who recovered from serious addictions without help. It examines the implications for drug abuse professionals and policymakers of recovery without treatment.

Stanton Peele's *The Meaning of Addiction: An Unconventional View* (reprint; San Francisco: Jossey-Bass, 1998) is one of the most insightful commentaries on addictive behavior. See also Chapter 7 of Andrew Weil's *Natural Health, Natural Medicine: A Complete Guide to Wellness and Self-Care for Optimum Health* (revised edition; Boston: Houghton Mifflin, 2004).

Some insight into the dangers of drug dealing and smuggling is provided by two entertaining books of true-life adventure: Robert Sabbag's *Snowblind: A Brief Career in the Cocaine Trade* (reprint; New York: Grove Press, 1998) and Bruce Porter's *BLOW: How a Small-Town Boy Made $100 Million with the Medellin Cocaine Cartel and Lost It All* (revised edition; New York: Griffin Trade Paperback, 2001). The latter was recently made into a popular movie. Another film, *Midnight Express,* is a horrifying story of the consequences of getting busted for drug smuggling abroad.

A readable history of our drug laws appears in *The American Disease: Origins of Narcotic Control* (third edition; New York: Oxford University Press, 1999) by David F. Musto, M.D. *Drug Control in a Free Society* by James B. Bakalar and Lester Grinspoon, M.D. (Cambridge: Cambridge University Press, 1988) is a balanced analysis of the arguments for and against various types of drug control.

13. Alternatives to Taking Drugs

A S WE MENTIONED at the beginning of this book, the main reason that people take psychoactive drugs is to satisfy a basic human need to vary their normal experience. Even very young children seem to have this need and experiment with techniques for altering their conscious state. Why should changing consciousness be so attractive and what do drugs have to do with it?

People who learn to change their conscious experience in safe and positive ways seem to be the better for it. They are healthier physically and mentally, more creative and productive, contribute more to society, and are more fun to be around. We believe that a desire to explore the various facets of consciousness is normal and good, but we are concerned about how people do it.

Being high does not mean being drugged. Clearly, drugs can sometimes make people feel high — at their best, energized, whole, expansive, creative, and connected. But why is it that many persons achieve high states without ever taking drugs, and why do the people who take the most drugs lose the very effects that they seek? The answer is that *drugs do not contain highs.* Highs exist within the human nervous system; all drugs do is trigger highs or provide an excuse to notice them.

That people cannot feel high whenever they want is one of the curious frustrations of the human condition. It seems necessary to work for highs or to find tools outside ourselves to evoke them. Drugs do this by making people feel temporarily different. They directly affect the nervous system and physical body in obvious ways. For example, stimulants make people feel wakeful and energized, and psychedelics alter body sensations and perceptions. Different drugs have different pharmacological effects, which is why they make people feel different in different ways.

No drug makes a person high automatically. One must learn to interpret the physical effects of drugs as the occasion for a high. It is expectations of individuals and society (set and setting) that encourage people to associate inner experiences with the physical feelings that drugs produce. If this association fails to develop or breaks down, people can take the largest imaginable doses of drugs and not get high — just feel drugged. This is precisely the problem of those who get into bad relationships with drugs by taking them too frequently: as the novelty of the drug's effect diminishes with repetition, it no longer produces the needed signal. First experiences are powerful because the novelty of the change is greatest.

It is very easy to confuse the signal with the desired experience, the drug with the high. Many drug users are convinced that the experiences that they need and like come from outside themselves in the form of drinks, joints, pills, and powders. It is this confusion that leads people to abuse drugs; they take more drugs more frequently in pursuit of ever-vanishing highs.

The fact that highs exist within is a cause for optimism. It means that the potential for these states is always there and many techniques must exist for eliciting them. There really *are* alternatives to drugs, because drug highs differ from other highs only in superficial ways. One day, scientists will understand what goes on in the brain when people feel high. It may be that these states are actually mediated by the brain's own neurochemicals, which can be stimulated equally by many different influences, including one's own thoughts. Everyone has had the experience of being rocketed out of a gloomy state by a word of praise, a demonstration of affection, or the arrival of a check in the mail. That change in mood might be exactly the same on the cellular level as the rapid euphoria that follows a snort of cocaine. In fact, it might not be accurate to talk about "natural" highs as opposed to "drug" highs, since both may depend on the body's endogenous drugs.

Is it any better to get high without drugs than with them? The main advantage of drugs compared to other techniques is that they work powerfully and immediately. *Their main disadvantage is that they reinforce the notion that the state that we desire comes from something outside us.* Not only can this idea lead to trouble with drugs, but it can also make people feel inadequate and incomplete. Even those in the best relationships with drugs often feel some degree of guilt about relying on them. Perhaps this feeling is so common because most people doubt their own worth and fear their abilities are not sufficient to meet the demands of life. Needing drugs to feel high confirms such fears. In any case, feeling guilty can't be good.

Of course, nondrug highs can present the same problem. People who are dependent on falling in love are equally at the mercy of outside forces. Many individuals get a rush from making money, and their lives are consumed in its pursuit. One variation on this theme is addiction to gambling. We have seen fanatical joggers who experience severe mental and physical discomfort if circumstances prevent them from running for even a day — a kind of withdrawal syndrome painful to them and those around them. If the only effective way you have of getting high is downhill skiing or hang-gliding, you are going to have to spend as much time and money getting high as any serious drug user and will expose yourself to equal or greater physical risk. There are men who get their greatest highs from killing; some of them find acceptable roles in society as professional soldiers, whereas others become criminals and terrorists.

The goal should be to learn how to get high in ways that do not hurt you or others and that do not necessarily require huge expenditures of time or money for special materials and equipment. Furthermore, you should be able to get high in enough different ways so that you can have the experience wherever you are, even if your external resources are minimal. You should also be willing to experiment with new methods of getting high as you mature and change.

Meditation, chanting, prayer, communing with nature, playing music, and artistic expression of all sorts are especially attractive ways of changing consciousness because they require little outside oneself. This is not to say that you shouldn't play polo if playing polo gets you high, but it would be useful to have some simpler, cheaper method in your repertoire as well.

Ways of changing consciousness without drugs do not work as fast or as powerfully as popping a pill; to master them, you may have to invest some time and effort. Many people may have little motivation to acquire these skills, especially since society neither admits the value of other modes of consciousness nor teaches us practical ways to achieve them. People who use drugs regularly may have to work especially hard to get high in other ways, because they often grow accustomed to the physical sensations of their drugs and consider them necessary components of the experience. People who use dilute forms of drugs infrequently and by mouth will find it easier to appreciate more subtle changes than people who put more concentrated drugs into their body more directly and more often, because they will not have learned to identify highs with intense pharmacological effects.

If getting high by simple methods takes more initial work, it may be worth it in the long run, because the simple methods do not fail with repeated use. In fact, methods requiring no external aid become more effective with practice. People who exercise, meditate, or do yoga to get high usually report that their experiences get better and better over time, which is a great contrast to the reports of heavy users of drugs.

There are so many ways to change consciousness that it is not worth trying to list them. Methods that work for some people may leave others cold. We know people who have learned to get high through Sufi dancing — a grown-up version of the spinning that children love — and others who find that this produces nothing

> Speaking in tongues makes me high. It makes me experi-
> ence an altered state of consciousness. It lets me glimpse
> another reality — infinite realities — beyond the scope of
> my "normal" state of consciousness.
>
> — thirty-year-old woman

more than motion sickness. Contact sports give some people terrific highs but offend the sensibilities of others. Some methods may
have more followers or seem more glamorous, but the only issue
of any importance is whether they work for you.

As we have noted, people also take drugs for reasons other than
getting high, and alternatives exist for these reasons as well. For
instance, it isn't necessary to take drugs to treat disease; many
drugless systems of therapy exist, such as acupuncture, massage,
and regulation of diet. Moods can be altered and performance improved by changing patterns of eating, sleeping, and exercise. Creativity can be stimulated by traveling, reading books, talking to
people, and having new experiences. You can explore your mind
with the aid of psychotherapy, hypnosis, or writing or singing
about your inner experiences. Since the use of drugs has become
so habitual in connection with certain activities (a glass of wine
with dinner, a joint before a movie), it may be hard for some people to imagine life without them. The fact is, however, that if people are determined enough, they can eliminate drugs from their
lives and never miss them.

SUGGESTED READING

For all of the talk about alternatives to drugs, precious little is in
print on the subject.

One of the best books is *Natural Highs: Supplements, Nutrition, and
Mind-Body Techniques to Help You Feel Good All the Time* by Hyla Cass
and Patrick Holford (New York: Avery Penguin Putnam, 2002).

Mind Games: The Guide to Inner Space by Robert Masters and Jean Houston (New York: Quest, 1998) is a manual of exercises in guided fantasy and trance states. The authors have written extensively about psychedelic experiences and are well qualified to discuss altered states of consciousness.

Originally published in 1968, *The Master Game: Pathways to Higher Consciousness* by Robert S. De Ropp and Iven B. Lourie (Nevada City, Calif.: Gateways Books & Tapes, 2003) remains an excellent book and practical guide.

Finally, Andrew Weil's *The Marriage of the Sun and Moon: Dispatches from the Frontiers of Consciousness* (revised edition; Boston: Houghton Mifflin, 2004) gives firsthand accounts of various nondrug highs and points out their relationship to drug experiences.

14. Final Words

SOME PEOPLE MIGHT THINK that giving the information in this book to young people will encourage them to try or to use drugs. We would like to address that question head-on.

The truth about drugs cannot do harm. It may offend some people's sensibilities and disturb those who do not want to hear it, but it cannot hurt people. On the other hand, false information can and does lead people to hurt themselves and others.

Our intention is not to encourage drug use by anyone, nor is it to discourage drug use. As we wrote at the very beginning, young people (and adults, for that matter) must decide for themselves which drugs, if any, to use and which to reject. We strongly recommend adopting alternatives to drugs, and we strongly recommend learning to use drugs wisely rather than falling into habits of excess, dependence, and abuse.

People make decisions on the basis of the information available to them. The more accurate the information, the better their decisions will be. We have worked hard to present balanced information that is as accurate as our best efforts can determine. We have not tried to make any drug attractive in our selection of facts.

If we have played down concerns about some drugs — say, the health hazards of marijuana — we have done so because they are products of bias and not in accord with our experience or compatible with the results of good scientific inquiry. In the end, such exaggeration of the dangers of marijuana leads more people to try the drug and more people to abuse it. We have countered those misconceptions by emphasizing what we see as a real danger of marijuana: the ease of sliding into a dependent relationship with it by smoking it thoughtlessly and excessively.

If we have stressed the ill effects of accepted drugs — say, those of coffee or antihistamines — we have done so because the findings about them are in accord with good scientific evidence and with our experience, and because we worry that ignorance of these hazards results in widespread overuse with attendant consequences on physical and mental health.

In short, we sincerely believe that the information that we have presented in these pages is reliable and will enable people to make intelligent choices about the use of drugs, which should help to prevent drug abuse before it starts.

Permit us to repeat the most important points that we have made:

There are no good or bad drugs, only good and bad uses of drugs. Drug abuse is not any use of a disapproved substance; abuse is the use of any substance in ways that impair physical or mental health or social functioning and productivity. Abuse develops from bad relationships with drugs, and learning to recognize such relationships early is one key to preventing abuse. Bad relationships with drugs begin with ignorance or loss of awareness of the nature of a substance and its effects and overuse of it to the point of losing the initial desired effect. Overuse, in turn, leads to difficulty in leaving the drug alone and to eventual impairment of health and productivity.

People must learn to look at and analyze their own and others' relationships with drugs. Recognizing drug abuse is not a matter of searching a child's room for cigarette papers or looking for dilated eyes or certain styles of dress or types of behavior. It involves the ability to know dependence in oneself and others, to watch how experiences with drugs change over time, to observe changes in health and look for correlations with drug use, to see whether drug usage interferes with work at school or on the job, to see whether it promotes associations with undesirable people. This kind of analysis is a lot harder than searching a room for cigarette papers.

Learning to recognize drug abuse is important, because treatment is not easy, and the earlier a problem comes to light, the better chance there is of correcting it. Prevention of drug abuse is always much easier than treatment. As we have said before, prevention depends on being informed, being aware, and exploring alternatives to drugs. For those who decide to use drugs, prevention depends also on associating with people who use drugs wisely rather than with people who abuse them, and on making intelligent choices about what substances to use and how and when to use them.

Treatment is another matter. Even with the best help possible, the only alternative for many abusers is to give up their drugs forever and admit that they have lost the chance to be in good relationships with those substances. In any case, treatment must begin with an abuser's own recognition that abuse exists and is a problem, and it will depend for its success on the individual's motivation to change. (Alcoholics Anonymous, Overeaters Anonymous, and other such self-help groups take this same position.) A drug abuser who is insufficiently motivated will not be cured by any approach.

Treating addiction often requires outside help: from doctors, counselors, clergy, and other professionals trained to advise people in trouble. Finding help is rarely easy, since some of the people most eager to work with drug abusers are in no way qualified to do the job. Above all, never put yourself or a child, relative, or friend in treatment for a drug problem with anyone you do not trust or consider fully informed and qualified, no matter what degree or certification the person holds.

Drug-abuse treatment centers are often staffed by ex-addicts. Such counselors may not be the best people to go to for help in improving your relationship with drugs, since they failed to form good ones themselves. Many reformed abusers behave like self-righteous fanatics when they appear in public: they inflame discussions about drugs, polarize audiences, and obstruct the drug-education process. It is also worth considering that the drug-abuse treatment profession has a vested interest in seeing drug abuse continue; its members make their living from the problem.

It is uncertain whether going to doctors for help is the best course of action. Medical schools do not teach much about the effects of psychoactive drugs. Unless physicians take the trouble to inform themselves, they are as likely as others to propagate untruths. Doctors have caused a great deal of the drug abuse of the past hundred years by carelessly prescribing opiates, cocaine, amphetamines, and tranquilizers without having clear ideas of the nature of those substances. Also, doctors themselves may be in bad relationships with alcohol, tobacco, coffee, and other depressants and stimulants legally available to them.

In sum, finding reliable help with drug problems is not simple. You have to shop around, ask questions, and use your own judgment. Do not hesitate to ask a prospective counselor to explain to you his or her attitudes toward drugs and recommendations for treatment of abuse. If you agree with the ideas in these pages, you might ask the person to read this book as a basis for your initial discussions.

If all of our warnings and cautions sound discouraging, it is because the treatment of drug abuse is discouraging. For that reason, we stress prevention as the better course and come back to solid, truthful information about drugs as the single best measure.

Suggested Reading lists follow most chapters, and we urge you to use them as a guide if you require more detail on a particular subject. The more you inform yourself on the complicated and ever-present issue of drugs, the more you can protect yourself and those around you from trouble, and the more you will be doing your part to steer society onto a less destructive course.

APPENDIX:

FIRST-PERSON ACCOUNTS

AND COMMENTS

GLOSSARY

INDEX

Appendix: First-Person Accounts and Comments

Drugs in High School A lot of kids in my high school were into drugs. The upperclassmen — myself included — smoked pot regularly and drank (mostly beer) on the weekends. The big status drug was cocaine, only no one could ever afford it. There was one kid who used to steal it from his parents, though, a little every day, and save it up for parties.

The main reason most kids took drugs — in my opinion — was peer pressure. Of course, we didn't admit that to ourselves. We weren't even conscious of it, really. It wasn't too obvious; if it had been obvious, it probably would have been a lot easier to resist. But it was a subtle thing, an attitude. We didn't think about it, but it was there.

— **twenty-eight-year-old man, carpenter**

The Coffee Cantata Johann Sebastian Bach (1685–1750) wrote the Coffee Cantata around 1732, when the new drink began to leave the male society of coffee houses in Germany and invade private homes, where ladies began to consume it. In the cantata, the father is angry because his daughter is a coffee addict. He threatens not to provide her with a husband unless she promises to stop drinking it. Here are a few excerpts from their dialogue:

FATHER: O wicked child! Ungrateful daughter, why will you not respect my wishes and cease this coffee drinking?

DAUGHTER: Dear Father, be not so unkind; I love my cup of coffee at least three times a day, and if this pleasure you deny me, what else on earth is there to live for?

DAUGHTER [continues in solo aria]: Far beyond all other pleasures, rarer than jewels or treasures, sweeter than grape from the vine. Yes! Yes! Greatest of pleasures! Coffee, coffee, how I love its flavor, and if you would win my favor, yes! Yes! let me have coffee, let me have my coffee strong.

FATHER: Well, pretty daughter, you must choose. If sense of duty you have none, then I must try another way. My patience is well nigh exhausted! Now listen! From your dress allowance I will take one half. Your next birthday should soon be here; no present will you get from me.

DAUGHTER: . . . how cruel! But I will forgive you and consolation find in coffee . . .

FATHER: Now, hearken to my last word. If coffee you must have, then a husband you shall not have.

DAUGHTER: O father! O horror! Not a husband?

FATHER: I swear it, and I mean it too.

DAUGHTER: O harsh decree! O cruel choice, between a husband and my joy. I'll strive no more; my coffee I surrender.

FATHER: At last you have regained your senses. [The daughter sings a melancholy aria of resignation.]

TENOR: And now, behold the happy father as forth he goes in search of a husband, rich and handsome, for his daughter. But the crafty little maiden has quite made up her mind that, ere she gives consent to marriage, her lover must make a solemn promise that she may have her coffee whenever and wherever she pleases.

Coffee Has Never Failed Me   In the morning I drink two cups of coffee. If I don't, I feel irritable. If I drink three cups, I get a little speedy, but with two I feel just about right.

If I drink coffee after about three in the afternoon, I cannot fall asleep when I like to, about eleven-thirty. If I drink coffee after dinner, as little as a half cup, I lie awake long past midnight. If I have something important or risky to do the next day, especially some public performance, coffee late in the day invariably interacts with my nervousness to produce stark insomnia.

This sleeplessness after coffee feels pharmacological. I can reach a dreamy peacefulness and experience some of the floating state that usually precedes sleep for me, but then I just hang on the edge, never quite slipping into unconsciousness. When I get up the next morning (angry at myself for not having slept), I feel relaxed but not rested by my seven hours in bed.

When I know that I have a long drive ahead of me, one that will mean driving late into the night or straight through it, I don't drink coffee for two or three days before. (I settle for lower doses of caffeine in tea or cola.) On the night of the drive I drink coffee twice, first a cup or two when I get drowsy at my usual bedtime, then two cups or more about three hours later. If I have been drinking coffee steadily for the few days before, I seem to get less stimulant effect from drinking it at night. It is almost a matter of "saving up" the coffee I would have consumed on the two or three days preceding and then drinking it on a particular night to keep me awake on the road. Used in this way, coffee has been a great help to me and has never failed me.

— **thirty-nine-year-old man, college administrator**

Coffee Addiction   My wife and I have drunk a lot of coffee for many years. I used to be a cigarette smoker but stopped with great difficulty twelve years ago; she still smokes, and I don't think she will ever be able to stop. I begin the day with two cups of coffee and drink about six more cups until dinnertime. Recently, we started drinking decaffeinated coffee with dinner, because we found the regular kind made it hard for us to fall asleep at bedtime.

A few years ago, I developed a shake in my left hand. The doctors call it a tremor and have no explanation or treatment for it. In the past year, it got worse and made me self-conscious. A number of people told me that caffeine might be causing it or, at least, making it worse, so I thought it would be a good idea to cut it out. Since I never thought that coffee did much for me or was much of a drug, I never thought it would be hard for me to stop.

My wife also thought of coffee as just a pleasant drink that we liked, and she agreed that we should switch to decaffeinated completely. So we did. I didn't notice any difference the first day, but on the second day I got very tired at my office and started to get a bad headache. I decided to come home early. When I arrived, I found my wife lying on the couch groaning. She said she had one of the worst headaches of her life and couldn't even stand up. Since my headache was steadily getting worse, I realized we must be experiencing a reaction to lack of caffeine. I told my wife that, but she refused to believe me. I told her I would prove it. I went to the kitchen and fixed us both cups of strong regular coffee. Within ten minutes of drinking them, we both felt our headaches disappear as if by magic and felt like our old selves. It astonished me to see how addicted we were to caffeine; my wife could scarcely believe it, since she was even less aware than I that coffee can be an addicting drug.

Since then, we have been trying to wean ourselves off caffeine by gradually substituting decaffeinated coffee for regular. We've cut our consumption in half so far but still cannot do without the two cups in the morning, even after a year of trying. We're determined to do it, however, and I know we'll succeed. Seeing the addiction for what it was gave us the motivation we needed.

— sixty-eight-year-old man, lawyer

Kicking the Chocolate Habit   Five years ago, hoping to kick a chocolate habit that was significantly affecting my life, I enrolled in a program at the Shick Center for the Control of Smoking, Alcoholism, and Overeating, in Los Angeles. I was then thirty-three. I could not remember the last time I had managed to get through a whole day without eating chocolate in one form or another, usually in quantities most people would regard as excessive, if not appalling.

Though not overweight, I indulged many of my chocolate cravings in secret, often in the middle of the night, when, if I had no chocolate in the house, I would think nothing of getting in my car and driving halfway across L.A. to an all-night supermarket for a fix. Although the Shick people told me they could cure my chocolate addiction in ten sessions, I was skeptical. My behavior was so compulsive and out of control that the best I thought I could hope for was a slight, temporary reduction of the cravings I suffered constantly. Still, I was willing to try anything.

The Shick Center places no importance on willpower, since it believes any form of self-imposed denial is doomed to failure. Instead, it uses a behavior-modification technique so simple as to seem ludicrous. Following instructions, I arrived for my first session with plenty of my favorite food (Hershey bars) and was seated in front of a mirror and handed a paper plate. A gadget was then strapped to my wrist that could give a very low-level electric shock. Far from being painful, this sensation was barely noticeable. I was told it was meant to have a purely subliminal effect. Thus equipped, I spent the next half-hour chewing mouthfuls of chocolate, which, instead of swallowing, I had to spit out onto the paper plate, all the while watching myself in the mirror.

During this first session, my skepticism hardened into utter disbelief. The mild revulsion I felt at the sight of seeing myself spit out the chocolate was more than offset by the pleasure of having it in my mouth. I couldn't see how such an absurd procedure could even scratch the surface of a problem as profound as mine, and were it not for the program's money-back guarantee, I would have dropped out then and there.

The following six sessions were carbon copies of the first. Toward the end of my seventh visit, I remember thinking, "This can't possibly be working; I still love the taste of chocolate as much as ever." Meanwhile, the program made no attempt to restrict what I ate on my own, and my chocolate consumption continued unabated.

It was not until the eighth session that I experienced a trace — it was the merest inkling — of something changing. It wasn't that I liked the taste of chocolate any less, but somehow I did not feel quite so compelled to put it in my mouth. Then, midway through the ninth session, I sensed a subtle but definite change. I didn't experience anything like distaste, but somehow eating the chocolate became automatic and without pleasure. I was still doubtful, especially about lasting effects, but the change was a revelation.

Preposterous as it may sound, I walked out of the tenth session completely cured. Although chocolate does not disgust me, I have no desire to eat it, ever. Flavors I never cared for before — vanilla, for example, or strawberry — appeal much more to me now, and I will choose them over chocolate every time. I don't consciously avoid chocolate out of fear of getting hooked again, either. I suppose I could get hooked again if I worked at it, but even though I test myself occasionally, my indifference to it remains the same.

Frankly, I am mystified by what happened and to this day cannot explain it. Being addicted to chocolate was so much a part of my definition of myself that it constantly amazes me to think that I am free of it. Needless to say, I am very grateful. The only problem is, I am now addicted (though somewhat less severely) to cake.

— **thirty-eight-year-old woman, social worker**

Trouble with Cocaine   I first tried cocaine in the early '70s. I had been using speed to help me with schoolwork and with my art. Cocaine was much more expensive than speed in those days and seemed less powerful, but I began to read a lot of information about the dangers of speed and thought cocaine might not be as harmful.

A few years later, I sold cocaine for a short time, although I still was not very involved with it. When I went to Europe on a vacation, I gave away what I had.

By the mid-70s, cocaine was more common, partly because the drug generation was older and had more money and partly because the dangers of speed were then well known. I found that coke gave me a good boost for getting work done. When I snorted it, I would feel inspired, brilliant, and energized. My art work went much faster with it because I could really focus on it and feel good at the same time. The ideas I got on coke were good ones, and I could get them down on paper. I came to see cocaine as an inducement and reward for getting work done.

Four years later, I began to realize that I could not work easily without cocaine. If I didn't use it, I felt bored, tired, and out of focus, which made me want to have it around all the time. As a result, I spent more and more money on it. I think I also began to get less patient, more critical, and paranoid. I started selling coke to friends to cover my needs, although I found dealing with friends as customers confusing and stressful. I got more and more difficult to be around. I was under a lot of work pressure, too, having to renovate a house I had acquired. I felt the need to rely on coke more and more to squeeze creative energy out of myself.

In 1978, a number of personal problems built up to an emotional crisis. A long-term love relationship broke up, and I ran into a dry spell with my art. I turned even more to coke to sustain me during this period. At first, a gram might last me a week, but soon I was using half a gram to a gram every day, sometimes having the first snort as soon as I got up. I would go for days without sleep. Also, I paid little attention to my diet. At one point, I had to go to the hospital with severe pain that turned out to be a kidney stone. I think it resulted from episodes of bad dehydration, since coke made me urinate more, but I would put off getting something to drink for hours while I buried myself in work.

In order to relax while using cocaine so heavily, I had to drink alcohol or take Valium. Even so, I would often lie in bed for hours with my heart racing, unable to fall asleep. I was really living in the extremes — either groggy and depressed or speeding. Finally, all that coke made me crazy. It gave me false inspiration and a kind of tunnel vision that hurt my creative efforts. Also, I began to suffer severe depressions. I'd play hide-and-seek games with the coke, locking it away and telling myself I wouldn't use it today. But as long as I knew it was there, I couldn't stop thinking about it and finally would give in and use it. Then I'd feel guilty as well.

I finally stopped taking it because the depressions outweighed the highs. After a few months, I tried it again but got the same results: depression and no high. I never again used cocaine, but I missed it for several years and had to relearn how to work without it. I feel strongly that I have to avoid any contact with that drug from now on.

— **forty-eight-year-old man, artist**

Speeding Through European History I was miserable and homesick during my first year at college and, as a result, wasn't a particularly good student. In fact, I spent the better part of my time bad-mouthing the school and sitting around feeling sorry for myself, and very little time studying. Therefore, when midterms came around, I had little hope of distinguishing myself. I decided to try and make up for lost time by staying up all night to study for my European history exam, but by midnight the text was blurring before my eyes. I was studying in the dining room of my dorm with several other girls. Seeing me losing my struggle to stay awake, an upperclassman took pity on me and offered me a green-and-white capsule along with the promise that my drowsiness would be cured by taking it. I took it without a second thought, and within half an hour or so found myself studying like mad. Not only was I completely engrossed in European history, I felt exhilarated; I was actually enjoying myself for the first time in months.

You always hear stories about people taking exams on amphetamines and thinking they've done brilliantly, only to find out later that they wrote page after page of incomprehensible gibberish. I almost wish that had happened in my case. I got an A on my history exam — as I was sure I had — and have been involved, to some extent, with amphetamines ever since.

— **forty-eight-year-old woman, writer**

A College Speed Freak I was a speed freak in college but did not know it, because a doctor got me to take it and never told me I could get hooked. I was about thirty pounds overweight and had never been able to diet for long. A school doctor started me on daily doses of Desoxyn and told me it would suppress my appetite. It did. It also made me feel great, at least at first. He also gave me a diet to follow, and I soon lost most of my excess weight. After several months, however, I began getting irritable and depressed and also didn't sleep well. I ate more when I was in these moods and gained some weight back. I found that taking more Desoxyn made me feel better and eat less.

It never occurred to me that the Desoxyn could affect my mood. I was completely ignorant of what it was; I think I considered it a kind of dietary supplement that took away hunger. My doctor never made me feel I needed to worry about taking it all the time. Soon, I was taking three times the original dose.

Even when speed began to get a bad reputation in the late 1960s, I didn't know I was on it. I was really shocked to learn that Desoxyn was just a brand name for methamphetamine and even more shocked to find that I couldn't stop taking it. If I tried to cut down the dose or stop, I would be groggy, depressed, and unable to concentrate or do my schoolwork. I would also eat a lot and gain weight. By the way, I also drank a lot of coffee and smoked cigarettes, so I was really a heavy user of stimulants.

When I told the doctor I was worried about being addicted, he made light of my fears, saying Desoxyn was a safe drug. It took many visits over the next year to convince him that I had a drug problem and took me another year beyond that to get off speed entirely. When I did, I was back where I started as far as being overweight. I feel I was a victim of that doctor's ignorance and probably of the drug company's promotion of the stuff for weight loss. Also, I know I was not an unusual case, because I have met other people who had similar experiences. I do not think I will ever take any kind of amphetamine again, because I am afraid that I would easily fall back into the same pattern of addictive use. Maybe those drugs have some good uses but not in the way I took them.

— **forty-six-year-old man, lawyer**

Speed in College: Another View   As a college student in the 1960s, I used speed to take important exams. Caffeine never helped me stay up; I could drink all the coffee I could stand or take many times the recommended dose of No-Doz and still fall asleep. So I went to the student health services, where a doctor listened to my story of getting sleepy when I had to study. He gave me a prescription for Dexamyl. The first time I took the stuff, I felt so good that I wrote a paper for a course effortlessly. I took another capsule the next day and got about half the effect. That made me realize I should not use it regularly.

The pattern I developed was to save the speed for the day of a big morning exam. I'd stay up studying as late as I could — say, till 3 A.M. — then go to sleep and set the alarm for seven. When I woke up, I'd study a little more and take a Dexamyl capsule when I left my room to walk to the exam. By the time I got the questions, I'd be buzzing with energy and confidence and be eager to start writing.

I did well in all the exams I took that way and never got any complaints that I'd written my name over and over. For me, Dexamyl really increased concentration and mental performance. (Of course, I had to know the material; it didn't put information in my head if I did not study.)

After I had made several visits to the student health service for new prescriptions, the doctor gave me an unlimited one that I used for several years, and [it] enabled me to give Dexamyl to classmates who also needed it at exam time. I never used speed in any other situations, and no one I knew in college had problems with it. I suppose that kind of prescription is not allowed anymore, and I know amphetamines have a bad reputation today, but I think we used them sensibly, and they helped us cope with a system that paralyzed many students with anxiety.

— **forty-nine-year-old man, corporate executive**

What I Think About Crank   Who would've thought my little town on the prairie would become the methamphetamine capital of the state? But it seems to be true. At least, the newspapers are full of stories about meth labs being raided and blowing up all over the county. Things are pretty bad around here. Family farms are going down the tubes, a lot of places on Main Street are boarded up, and most people who could move away have moved away. I know a few people who take crank to drive at night or do housework, but I've never run into any hardcore addicts. Meanwhile, just about every kid is on speed for ADD [attention deficit disorder]. Imagine my surprise when I found out that the most popular prescription drug for kids around here is Adderall, which is — guess what? — methamphetamine. It seems to me something is wrong with this picture.

— **twenty-nine year-old woman, beautician**

A Nonaddicted Smoker   Like Mark Twain, I find it easy to give up smoking; I have done it countless times. In fact, I consider myself a nonaddicted smoker, since I have been smoking cigarettes on and off for twenty-five years without ever getting so hooked I couldn't stop just like *that* whenever I chose to. I would see nothing extraordinary about this, were it not for the wonder and admiration it excites in other people. Since it is mostly unheard of to smoke cigarettes only now and then, acquaintances regard me as a woman of superhuman willpower, a notion I hate to disabuse them of.

However, the sad truth is, I have no more willpower than anyone else and probably less than many. What saves me from being a cigarette junkie is that I recognized early how easy it would be for me to get hooked on tobacco, and, knowing that if I did get hooked I'd hate myself, I have always been very careful to keep my smoking under control.

For one thing, I never smoke before five o'clock in the afternoon. That, in itself, might seem adequate insurance against addiction, but, even though I have no desire for a cigarette before that time, I have been known to smoke up to five in a row once I begin — making myself very sick in the process. So I limit myself to one cigarette before dinner and try not to smoke more than five or six in the course of an evening. Also, I monitor my consumption very closely, and whenever I notice a rising trend, I swear off entirely for a few days.

Since my husband is a confirmed and heavy smoker, it requires some effort on my part to refrain entirely for days at a time. On the other hand, having him around helps me in the long run because he provides a living example of the sort of dependency I want so much to avoid.

— **thirty-seven-year-old woman**

Love versus Cigarettes   These days I run into lots of people who have stopped smoking, and they always say, "You could do it, too." I suppose they're right in theory. I mean, in theory I could run the triathalon if I put my mind to it, but in practice I know it isn't so.

I come from a long line of smokers. At seventy, my mother still smokes heavily. Her mother smoked well into her eighties (and lived to be ninety-three). I took up the habit at age thirteen, and for the next twenty years I never once seriously considered denying myself the pleasure [that] smoking afforded me.

Then, several years ago, I fell madly in love with an ex-smoker, a man who, though broad-minded in other respects, was a fanatic on the subject of cigarettes. He forbade smoking anywhere in his vicinity — not only in his own house and car but also in other people's houses and cars, as well as in restaurants and movie theaters, where he would not hesitate to browbeat people into putting out their cigarettes even when they were legally within their rights to smoke.

Very early in our relationship, I realized it would be futile to expect him to compromise on this issue. Not only did he object to cigarette smoke in the air he breathed, he hated the smell of it on my breath, in my hair or clothing. He was also highly sensitive to the odor of cigarettes, and though I bent over backwards to avoid offending him, my efforts were mostly unsuccessful. I grew increasingly defensive and insecure, and soon had to face the fact that we couldn't possibly have a long-term, intimate relationship unless I quit smoking. I therefore resolved to do so, and one day, feeling very virtuous, I tossed out my cigarettes and went cold turkey.

My friend assured me that I would soon begin to feel great as a result of not smoking, but in fact the discomfort I experienced from abstinence was intense and unrelenting, even after five weeks. Smoking had become so woven into the fabric of my life that everything seemed to come unraveled without it. I could not get my mind off cigarettes for more than ten seconds at a time. I craved them not only every minute of every day but also in my dreams at night.

Naturally, my agony put a lot of stress on what was still an untried and untested relationship, and the relationship did not bear up well under it, I'm afraid. No doubt, I wanted much more credit and consideration from my friend than I deserved, but I also deserved, I think, somewhat more than I got. Having gone through the ordeal himself, he was, if anything, less compassionate. He did not want to hear about my suffering and put me down for continuing to make such a fuss. Then, after five weeks of steadily mounting tension, he had to go to Europe on business for a month. I started smoking again as soon as his plane took off.

When my friend returned from Europe, he was most unhappy to find that instead of being out of the woods, I was right back at square one. He was willing to try again, but this time, instead of urging me to quit for reasons of my own health and well-being, he wanted me to do it for him. What meant more to me — him or cigarettes? That was the choice I was faced with. In other words, it was a test.

Well, to make a long story short, I failed the test — not once or twice but repeatedly, almost every day for ten straight months, in fact. Had my lapses been matters merely between me and my conscience, they would have been bad enough. But, as I said, my friend was very sensitive to the odor of tobacco. No matter what precautions I took, he was able, even hours after the fact, to smell the evidence on my breath. So I was constantly humiliated as well, and my failures became the subject of endless arguments, and, toward the end of the affair, the cause of several knock-down, drag-out fights. There were, of course, other differences between us, but the issue of smoking became a sort of lightning rod, attracting more and more of the emotional charge.

I had always thought I'd be able to kick my addiction for someone I loved. That assumption turned out to be wrong. In the end, when forced to choose between love and cigarettes, I chose cigarettes. It was that simple.

I did make one resolution at the time, which I have stuck to ever since. It was that I would never again become involved with a man who does not smoke cigarettes.

— **forty-one-year-old woman, teacher**

I Like Alcohol   I like alcohol. It is a powerful drug and, God knows, for some people a hellish one, but if used carefully it can give great pleasure. After a long, hard day, the splendid warm glow that strong drink provides is one of my favorite feelings; it starts in the pit of my stomach, then spreads to my limbs and brain. I know that alcohol is a depressant, but it acts and feels like a gentle relaxant — of the spirit as well as of the physical body. Just notice the increased vivacity and noise level at a cocktail party after a drink has been served to see how alcohol can put people at ease emotionally.

Aside from the pleasureful intoxication of strong drink, I also enjoy the tastes of lighter forms of alcohol. Few sensations are more delightful than the wet but dry taste of cold beer to a parched throat. The subtle, taste-enhancing, enriching relationship of wine to food is a subject that has inspired many poets and writers far more capable than I of putting words together, but I can tell you that what they say is true. The fascinating, complex flavor of good wine can be profoundly sensual.

— **sixty-two-year-old man, psychoanalyst**

Bad Drinking Habits   I was sixteen when I first got drunk. It was a revelation, more fun than a barrel of monkeys. I screamed and hollered and carried on and did somersaults and hugged my friends (who were also drunk) and just had a blast. Naturally, I kept wanting to repeat the experience.

Pretty soon, a group of my high-school friends and I got into regular weekend parties where we'd get drunk (usually on hard liquor) and lose our inhibitions. Sometimes we'd even bring a bottle to school and sneak out between classes to drink a little. No one knew anything about pot or other drugs in those days. Alcohol was it. It was our main way of getting high and so was very important to us.

When I went away to college, I continued my pattern of using alcohol to get high, mostly at weekend parties. But two things began to happen that bothered me. First, from doing it over and over, the alcohol high lost a little of its fascination for me. Although I still liked it, it didn't measure up to those early experiences in high school. Secondly, I started getting bad hangovers. I mean, I'd really be sick as a dog the next day, and I didn't like that at all. The price seemed much too high to pay for a few hours of fun.

I used to tell myself I'd only drink to the point of getting pleasantly high, but every single time I'd go beyond it. Before I'd know it, I'd be stumbling around, being loud and jovial, insensitive to pain. I'd feel great at the time, and I'd also know what was in store for me. Usually, the sick effects would start when I'd try to go to sleep drunk: terrible nausea with the room spinning. Every serious drinker knows that one. And the next day, I'd be totally out of action, feeling as if I'd been poisoned, which I guess I had. I got really scared one time when I woke up like that and couldn't remember anything of the night before.

Although I kept trying to use alcohol moderately, whenever I'd set out to get high on it, I would always keep on drinking till I got drunk, no matter how many resolutions I made not to.

About that time, pot came along. It took me a little while to learn to get high on it, but when I did, it seemed much better than alcohol for me. There was no problem of taking too much and behaving badly, no getting sick, and no hangover. Becoming a pot smoker got me out of my bad drinking habits. I think if I'd kept them up, I would now be in real trouble.

I've tried various drugs since those days and don't think anything comes close to alcohol in terms of raw strength and potential for trouble. I couldn't learn to control it well, and I see many people around me who have the same problem.

— **thirty-seven-year-old man, college professor**

An Overdose of Downers   The old saying "The cobbler's children go without shoes" applies to the children of physicians, too. Because they deal with sick people all day long, doctors tend to give short shrift to the complaints of family members. As the daughter of a medical doctor, I should know. When I or any of my brothers or sisters came down with anything more serious than a hangnail, my father's standard procedure was to ply us with sleeping pills.

When I was very young, his prescription was for a half-grain or so of phenobarbital, but by the time I was in junior high school, whenever I had a sore throat or stuffy nose, I was sent to bed with two Seconals or Nembutals as a matter of course. The theory behind this treatment was that a good night's sleep would cure just about anything, and though it did not always work out that way, I never doubted the basic principle or questioned the wisdom of using drugs to implement it.

Later, when I was living on my own, my father gave me an assortment of sleeping pills to have on hand just in case. Falling asleep was never one of my problems, so I never resorted to them on my own. Then, one night when I had come down with a severe cold, my father stopped by and advised me to take some sedatives to be sure to get a good night's sleep. I said okay, produced the grab bag of pills, and asked him which to take. He chose two of the biggest gelatin capsules I had ever seen. They were Placidyl, he told me, 250 milligrams each. I protested, sure that one would more than do the job, but he insisted they were very mild, and that 500 milligrams was the standard dose. After I'd taken them, he left.

Meanwhile, I had been waiting for a neighbor to come and walk my dog in the park across the street. After twenty minutes or so, when she still hadn't arrived, I decided I'd take the dog out quickly myself. I was starting to feel groggy and wanted to go to sleep.

I lost consciousness almost as soon as I reached the street. All of a sudden, there was a fantastic explosion of lights, and I remember looking up at the sky, exclaiming "Wow!" before blacking out. That must have been around ten-thirty. When I came to, it was after midnight, and people were shaking me and slapping my face. I was in the park, where some other dog walkers had discovered me on a bench in a stupor. Apparently, the dog had dragged me in a somnambulent state all the way up the block, across a big street, and into the park. The people who found me had been slapping me for several minutes without success. Figuring I had either overdosed on something accidentally or made a suicide attempt, they were on the verge of calling an ambulance. It was obvious to everyone that I was heavily drugged, and, of course, they were all upset. When I realized what had happened, I was beside myself with rage.

Calling my father on the telephone to rant and rave brought no satisfaction. He not only refused to accept any responsibility for what had occurred — sticking to his story about 500 milligrams of Placidyl being a mild dose — he even tried to shift the blame onto me by suggesting that I had some deep, unconscious motive for passing out in the street. I hung up, consciously motivated to strangle him.

As it turned out, my father had given me not 500 milligrams of Placidyl but twice that amount: 1,000 milligrams, or, as the package insert put it, enough to knock out a woman in labor. Nevertheless, he continued to make light of the incident and deny any negligence on his part.

On the whole, the experience was very valuable for me because it taught me something people need to know — namely, that it is good to be skeptical about doctors (whether or not they are relatives) and the casual ways they dispense drugs.

— **thirty-eight-year-old woman, artist**

Experiences with Quaalude Many of my friends and I began using methaqualone, or Quaaludes, in the 1960s. We take them on occasion only and like the way they remove inhibitions and ease social interactions. I know a lot of folks who consider Quaalude their drug of choice, especially for having fun and partying.

I've seen Quaalude produce hilarious situations. One time I went with a group of friends to dinner at a fancy Italian restaurant. Most of us took Quaalude before leaving the house. We ordered dinner in high spirits and, when it came, started eating. Just then, one woman who had taken a double dose passed out and fell face first into her plate of spaghetti. Everyone else stood up and applauded.

I've also seen Quaalude lead to tragic situations. Everyone knows that downers and driving don't mix. I know a woman who was trying to cope with severe depression by taking Quaalude. One night, after exceeding her usual dosage, she went out and almost lost her life in an auto accident. She ran into a parked car.

I've seen other people become violent on Quaalude, then not remember it afterwards — just as with alcohol. One man who saw me professionally told me he once took three Quaaludes and went to bed. The next thing he remembered was being awakened about two hours later by his frightened wife, who told him he had been beating her.

There is no question that Quaalude can be dangerous when used irresponsibly, or that it can be addicting. As a recreational drug, taken on occasion in a responsible manner, it seems to me safe and interesting and gives me an experience different from anything else.

One of the rules I follow is to know my tolerance so that I take the right dose. Black-market Quaaludes are more of a problem, because their quality is uncertain. Usually, they contain less methaqualone than pharmaceutical Quaaludes, but they really vary. I've seen two people with equal tolerance each take one black-market Quaalude and experience different effects. So knowing your drug is important, too.

The other rules that are most important are not to mix Quaalude with alcohol and not to mix Quaalude with driving.

— **forty-six-year-old man, drug counselor**

Down on Valium I hope I never hear of Valium again. A university physician gave it to me as a "muscle relaxant" when I had a pinched nerve in my neck that caused muscle spasms in my right shoulder and weakness in my right hand. He did not tell me anything about the mental effects of Valium, so I was quite unprepared for them. All I remember of the next few days is that I could not concentrate in my office. Then my secretary and wife began acting strange. Only when I stopped taking the drug did I realize how bizarre my behavior had become while I was on it. I would stare blankly into space when people talked to me, not remember anything said to me, and be unable to think or reason. Also, I had no sense that anything was wrong. I think Valium turned me into a kind of zombie for those few days. I can't understand why anyone would want to take it.

— **sixty-two-year-old man, university professor**

Valium as a Tool   I first began taking Valium ten years ago to relieve anxiety and very quickly came to depend on it for writing, or, more exactly, for beginning to write. Once I am at my desk and have actually begun to work, I am fine; the problem for me is to get there in the first place. What I discovered was that very soon after I took a dose of Valium, I felt high, and that during the brief period that the high lasted, getting to my desk was a whole lot easier.

By now, after ten years of experimenting, I have learned that, like any tool, Valium has its limitations. It works best on an empty stomach, for example, and when it comes to dosage, less is definitely more. Two and a half milligrams is the right dose for me; more than that makes me feel groggy. Also, since I become tolerant to its effects if I take it more than two days running, I have to use it intermittently.

Even when I observe all the rules and take Valium under ideal conditions, the period of grace it affords me is extremely brief. Once its effects begin to come on, I have about fifteen minutes in which to capitalize on them. During that critical period, if I happen to be distracted by a phone call or a neighbor dropping by, all is lost. That sounds hard to believe, I know, but it has happened to me many times, and whenever it does, that's it: the day is shot. Besides being too anxious to get to my desk, I will be furious — positively fit to be tied.

— **thirty-nine-year-old woman, writer**

GHB   GHB put me in a state unlike any I'd ever experienced before and would just as soon not experience again. It was given to me by a friend who was visiting for the weekend. We took it at about eleven P.M., after which my guest went off to bed. I continued tidying things up in the kitchen for maybe fifteen more minutes until, all of a sudden, I felt a wave of nausea and started to sweat. I decided to just stop what I was doing and go to bed. Well, I had already come to a stop, so that was no problem. The problem was that I could not go. I wanted to go, but I was not able to move. It felt as if there were a glitch in my automated equipment and I had to reach around and manually operate my brain. It required fierce concentration to advance even in super-slow motion, and concentrating made me sick to my stomach. Whenever I stopped, though, to let the nausea subside, I became paralyzed again, transfixed, until I somehow managed to summon up the will to resume the effort. Ordinarily, I can make the trip between the kitchen and my bedroom in less than thirty seconds. That night it took about a month.

— thirty-three-year-old woman, secretary

An Anesthetic Revelation   I once inhaled a pretty full dose of ether, with the determination to put on record, at the earliest moment of regaining consciousness, the thought I should find uppermost in my mind. The mighty music of the triumphal march into nothingness reverberated through my brain, and filled me with a sense of infinite possibilities, which made me an archangel for a moment. The veil of eternity was lifted. The one great truth which underlies all human experience and is the key to all the mysteries that philosophy has sought in vain to solve, flashed upon me in a sudden revelation. Henceforth all was clear: a few words had lifted my intelligence to the level of the knowledge of the cherubim. As my natural condition returned, I remembered my resolution; and, staggering to my desk, I wrote, in ill-shaped, straggling characters, the all-embracing truth still glimmering in my consciousness. The words were these (children may smile; the wise will ponder): "A strong smell of turpentine prevails throughout."

— Oliver Wendell Holmes (1809–1894), American physician
and author, from a lecture given in 1870

The Need for Opiates   The first opiate I ever took was codeine. I snorted it. It made me feel right for the first time in my life. I said to myself, "Aha, this is what I've been missing." I never felt right from as far back as I can remember, and I was always trying different ways to change how I felt. I used lots of drugs, including pot, downers, tranquilizers, and alcohol, but none of them ever really did it for me. Codeine was a revelation, and I've been an opiate user ever since.

That first time, I was twenty-three. Before long, I was addicted, although I've always snorted dope, never shot it. Opiates have caused me lots of trouble, but what they do for my head is worth it. Now I'm thirty-four and am on methadone maintenance. I don't think methadone is the best opiate for me; it makes me sweat terribly and has some other effects on my body I don't like, but it's great to be able to get what I need legally, so that I can spend time on things other than scoring. I hope one day more people will realize that some of us have to have opiates just to feel normal.

— **thirty-four-year-old woman, rock singer**

Opiate Addiction   I started using heroin in high school, chipped for a long time, then finally became an addict. Presently, I'm on methadone, which works well for me. I use narcotics to keep from feeling sick (withdrawal), to relieve stress, and sometimes for fun. I like to mainline because it's the most economical way to take opiates: heroin is at least three times as active intravenously as orally, although the effects last longer if you take it by mouth.

I've read a lot about opiate users' seeking a "rush" by injecting heroin. To me, the rush has never been that important. It feels like a pleasant warm feeling, especially in the pit of the stomach, accompanied by deep physical and mental relaxation. (Incidentally, smoking many opiates gives a stronger rush than mainlining, but it is wasteful, because some of the drug is destroyed by heat.) In my experience, chippers are more interested in rushes than addicts. They tend to take narcotics on occasion for fun, whereas addicts take them regularly in order to make it through a troubled world. Regular doses of heroin just make many addicts feel normal; they do not give noticeable rushes.

For me, the rush is secondary to the tranquilizing and pain-relieving effects of opiates. I feel I have a metabolic problem due to lack of endogenous opiate-like drugs. By substituting external narcotics for internal ones, I have probably shut off my body's production of the endogenous substances, and now I have to take opiates regularly to make life bearable. Sometimes I'll take a higher than usual dose for pleasure and savor the rush, but that's unusual. Oral methadone does not give a rush, and if rushes were so important to addicts, methadone maintenance would not be accepted by so many of them. As I've said, it works for me.

By the way, my health has been generally good since I've been an opiate addict. I don't get colds when other people do, and when I travel in

Mexico, I don't get dysentery, although my nonusing companions do, and we eat the same food.

— thirty-year-old man, chemist

LSD and Psilocybin I have been unable to identify any sign at all of addiction, organic injury, or other in some way unpleasant aftereffects . . . In my opinion, however, LSD and psilocybin cannot and should not become "pleasure drugs" for the general public. Their effects are such that they lead one beyond the customary (and constraining) coordinate system of space and time, and afford insights into the heaven and hell of one's own self — which can be dangerous to one who is not cut out for that, and hence is not prepared.

According to my experience, only several repeated experiments afford a serious appraisal. I also believe that at least one of these experiments should be undertaken in familiar surroundings (under discreet supervision of a trusted person) and with higher doses. *Only* then might the drug show us its, and our, deepest secret.

— Rudolf Gelpke, a Swiss professor of Islamic studies
who took LSD and psilocybin a number of times in 1961

A DMT Disaster The only time I ever took a psychedelic was a disaster. It was in the early 1960s, and the drug was DMT. I knew nothing about it. Some friends invited me to their place and told me they wanted to share a pleasant experience with me. They said they would inject a small amount of a new drug into my leg. It was safe and would give me a nice feeling for a short time. I agreed to try it.

Within a few minutes of the injection, I was swept into a nightmare world of horrible visions, such as finding myself wading into an ocean where all sorts of monsters attacked me. The real world disappeared so completely I thought I'd never see it again. Even years later, I can still recall the feeling of slimy tentacles grabbing my legs and trying to pull me underwater. When I came back from this frightening place, I was so shaken that I stayed in my room for two days. It took me a very long time to get over being afraid of the ocean afterwards, and to this day I have been unable to try another psychedelic, although I am curious about the good effects people have described to me. I think those friends who gave me DMT were not malicious, just irresponsible. I wonder how many others have had similar bad experiences from taking psychedelic drugs with no preparation?

— **thirty-five-year-old man, movie producer**

Peyote Visions My first vivid show of mescal colour effects came quickly. I saw the stars, and then, of a sudden, here and there delicate floating films of colour — usually delightful neutral purples and pinks. These came and went — now here, now there. Then an abrupt rush of countless points of white light swept across the field of view, as if the unseen millions of the Milky Way were to flow a sparkling river before the eye. In a minute this was over and the field was dark. Then I began to see zigzag lines of very bright colours . . .

When I opened my eyes all was gone at once. Closing them I began after a long interval to see for the first time definite objects associated with colours. The stars sparkled and passed away. A white spear of grey stone grew up to a huge height, and became a tall, richly finished Gothic tower of very elaborate and definite design, with many rather worn statues standing in the doorways or on stone brackets. As I gazed, every projecting angle, cornice, and even the faces of the stones at their joinings were by degrees covered or hung with clusters of what seemed to be huge precious stones, but uncut, some being more like masses of transparent fruit. These were green, purple, red, and orange; never clear yellow and never blue. All seemed to possess an interior light, and to give the faintest idea of the perfectly satisfying intensity and purity of these gorgeous colour-fruits is quite beyond my power. All the colours I have ever beheld are dull as compared to these.

— **from an essay by Dr. S. Weir Mitchell (1829–1914), an American physician and novelist who drank an extract of peyote in 1896**

I Smoked a Toad In August of 1990 I visited a friend of mine who lived in the desert near Tucson, Arizona. He is a long-time psychedelic tripper who mainly likes mushrooms and peyote. I once brought him some MDMA, but he refused to try it, saying he only took natural psychedelics. So when I got to his house, he told me he had a new favorite drug: toad venom. I thought he was kidding me, but he pulled out a vial that held small, transparent chips of what he said was dried venom he had collected from the big desert toads that come out at night during the summer rains. He showed me some of these guys during my visit; I never knew toads got so big. He also showed me how to handle them and get the venom to squirt out of the glands in their heads. Anyway, one night we smoked a chip of this stuff in a small pipe. It had a strong flavor. I took one toke and held it in for maybe fifteen seconds. By the time I exhaled, I felt like I was going up in an elevator to somewhere else. I was lying down in a desert wash, and it was a beautiful night, but I think I was just somewhere else for a while. When I became aware of my surroundings, I couldn't talk for a long time and felt that the sounds of the desert were vibrating in my body. It was very intense and very strange. After a few more minutes, I felt like myself again. Then I started laughing. It just struck me so funny that these big old toads could make you high. I'd like to see the feds try to go after them.

— **thirty-three-year-old man, massage therapist**

The Love Drugs   I first took MDA in 1970. I thought it was the most wonderful experience I ever had. I remember lying in a field with four good friends, just lying in a big hug pile for hours, not wanting anything to be different, totally content, completely in the here and now. I felt like a lion in a pride of lions on an African plain, totally secure in the physical closeness with my brothers and sisters. Over the next few years, I took MDA maybe three or four times a year, always with the same good results, but I did find there was a price to pay: I'd be nonfunctional for a day or two afterward.

When MDMA came along a few years later, I was delighted. It was legal, shorter acting, and the price I had to pay was much, much less, at least at first. I turned a lot of people on to it and saw it do incredible things: save marriages, create lifelong friendships, lead to people falling in love. One of my friends produced a T-shirt that said, "Don't Get Married for at Least Six Weeks After Ecstasy!" I think MDMA could put a lot of psychiatrists and psychologists out of business.

I wish I could still use MDMA once a month, as I used to, but I'm afraid that as I've gotten into middle age, I can't handle the burned-out feeling I get the next day. Even taking lower doses, I can barely drag myself around or focus my mind for the next twenty-four hours. So now I take it maybe once a year. I still think it's one of the best drugs ever invented.

— **fifty-one-year-old man, university professor**

Psychedelic Therapy   As a clinical psychologist who has treated hundreds of patients with psychedelic drugs over the past twenty-five years, I consider LSD, MDMA, magic mushrooms, mescaline, and the rest to be the most valuable therapeutic tools I know to show people how they can change in positive directions.

Because my use of these drugs is not approved under current laws or standards of practice, I cannot publish my findings or engage openly in psychedelic therapy. Still, I have trained many other psychiatrists and psychologists to use this method and have been able to treat many patients successfully. I am very careful in selecting patients for this kind of treatment, very careful in preparing them for a psychedelic session, in conducting the session, and in following it up with the kind of work that enables patients to make practical use of the insights they gain.

Conventional forms of psychotherapy often enable people to understand how their habits of thinking about themselves and others produce frustration and pain, but you can spend years in therapy gaining all this insight and keep on being the same frustrated, neurotic person. One good psychedelic session can make you *feel* what you are doing and show you how to do it differently. In the right hands and settings, these drugs can convince you that the worst problem in your life can be solved by changing your own attitudes and ways of perceiving and can motivate you to make the necessary changes.

It is a shame that more doctors and patients do not take advantage of this potential.

— seventy-year-old man, psychologist

The Day the Universe Ended: Salvinorin-A   I consider myself very experienced with psychedelics and was curious to try *Salvia divinorum*. I got a plant of it and was intending to smoke the leaves, but before I got a chance to do it, a friend came by and offered me some pure crystalline salvinorin-A. He put a little bit in a glass pipe, held a flame underneath, and told me to take one deep hit of the vapor. I did, and the next thing I knew, everything ended. I was reduced to a little spark of consciousness, suffocated and trapped by an immense weight. This was it. Eternity. And I kept hearing a malevolent cosmic laugh at my fate as well as a vision of that little pipe. It was as if all my life led up to the moment where I was offered the pipe. I had a choice. And I chose to inhale that vapor. And fall into the trap from which there was no escape. It was eternal imprisonment in a tiny cage with nothing, absolutely nothing, outside of it. I can't begin to convey the psychic discomfort I was in. Of course, at some point, maybe ten or fifteen minutes later, the effect of the drug subsided, and I got some perspective on what had happened. I suppose I took way too much. When I was able to stand up, the first thing I did was throw out the *Salvia divinorum* plant that had been on a window sill. Other people have told me they've had good experiences smoking the leaves, but I have no interest in trying them.

— **fifty-year-old man, computer scientist**

Quitting Pot   I smoked marijuana for about seven years, mostly during college and law school. It was great for me at first, a real relaxer and sense-enhancer, and I had a lot of good times with it. Occasionally, I had bad reactions to it — paranoia, shaking, pounding heartbeat, and feeling cold all over. Sometimes I'd have this reaction every time I'd smoke over a period of a week or so, then I wouldn't have it again for many months. I don't know what it came from, maybe being in uncomfortable environments or around people I didn't like.

Eventually, I became a daily pot smoker, sometimes starting in the morning. It was my main way of relating to other people. However, I started getting less and less effect from it that I liked. In fact, it began to make me groggy and sleepy most of the time and also gave me a cough. These unwelcome effects got worse and worse until I realized I would have to stop using pot. So I made a resolution to quit completely.

Well, it surprised me to find that wasn't so easy. It took me three years of trying before I really gave up smoking marijuana, even though I no longer got pleasant effects from it. I never realized how much of a habit I had and how hooked I was on it. I was certainly abusing the stuff. I think I'd better just stay off it for good now. I'm afraid that if I tried to use it once in a while, my smoking would just creep back up to that addictive level, and I'd be in the same spot as before.

I don't have bad feelings about pot. I learned a lot from it and never really got hurt by it. I think it should be legalized. I also think people who use it should be aware that it can have strong effects and can be addicting if you don't watch out.

— **forty-one-year-old man, lawyer**

Marijuana and Driving   You want to know about marijuana and driving? When I first tried driving when stoned, it was pretty weird. I would imagine I was cruising along at fifty miles per hour but would only be going twenty. Sometimes I'd feel as if I were very, very tiny behind a gigantic steering wheel. Going through a long tunnel, I thought I was driving vertically down a shaft into the earth. These illusions were both scary and fun. I never had an accident, but I'm a good driver to begin with and was always careful. I can see where pot could be dangerous for someone not used to it.

One time, while I was in college, I was very stoned late at night in Cleveland and had to drive home. I was going through deserted streets in residential neighborhoods. Suddenly, I couldn't remember whether I was in Cleveland or Pittsburgh, where I grew up. I could turn the scene through the window into either city. Then I came to an intersection that was very familiar, only I had to turn left if it was Cleveland and right if it was Pittsburgh. That's the kind of mind tricks pot can play on you at the wheel.

Later, when I had been smoking marijuana for several years, I never had such strong effects anymore, and driving after smoking was pretty routine for me. A number of times I almost had accidents because joints fell apart on me while I was driving or because lighting a pipe behind the wheel took my attention (and hands) off the wheel. Those hazards were more dangerous than direct effects of the drug.

Finally, pot started making me really sleepy and groggy a lot, and that was a problem for driving, especially when I was by myself on a long haul. I'd think, Boy, it would be nice to smoke a joint, this ride is really boring. So I'd light up and feel pleasantly high for ten minutes or so, then spend the next two hours fighting off the nods. It was no different from getting sleepy normally, but that sure is risky on an interstate highway for you and other people, if you don't pull off at a rest stop and either take a nap or somehow wake yourself up.

— **thirty-two-year-old man, lab technician**

Marijuana as Medicine   Twenty years ago, I suddenly developed a paralysis of the right side of my body that baffled the doctors. After ten months, it began to improve, but I also lost my vision and that came back only in part. They finally were able to make a diagnosis of multiple sclerosis.

About three years later, I discovered marijuana. A friend told me it was relaxing. My main problem then, aside from partial blindness, was tenseness and tremors in my muscles. Pot cured it, and I've smoked regularly ever since, about four to five times a week. If I go without it for a week, the muscle tremors come back.

Medical science has nothing to offer me. Most people with MS have repeated attacks and keep losing body function. I'm convinced that pot has kept me in remission all these years. It can't help my vision, because there was permanent nerve damage. Still, I can get around fairly well. It does keep my muscles in great shape. I lift weights regularly and feel pretty strong.

I can't believe that marijuana is not legally available for medical use, that a doctor can't prescribe it for me. I want to see it legalized, and I want the government to supply me with it. I'm a veteran and think I ought to get my pot from the VA hospital.

— **forty-one-year-old man, part-time roofer**

Dr. Mom My son, now eighteen, began getting splitting headaches when he was twelve. A year later, they finally got around to testing him for Lyme disease, he tested positive, and was treated with high doses of antibiotics intravenously. When he was cured, though, his headaches didn't go away. None of the myriad drugs that doctors recommended over the next couple of years did anything but cause all sorts of hideous so-called side effects. He was put on every drug that could conceivably be used to treat migraine headaches — Fiorinal, numerous prescription allergy medications, beta-blockers, calcium-blockers, Imitrex, you name it. Some were worse than others, but they were all bad — bad for your kidneys, your liver, et cetera. Reading the inserts used to drive me nuts. And it wasn't just drugs — we tried acupuncture, cranial manipulation, psychotherapy, biofeedback, homeopathy — and absolutely nothing worked.

I'm not sure when, but at some point, my son started smoking pot and it relieved his headaches. I'm not saying it got rid of them, but it *helped*. So I wasn't going to tell him not to use it. But I still kept taking him to doctors. Eventually, one day when he was in excruciating pain and didn't have any pot, I called a friend and got him some. In other words, I became a criminal. My son was the one who pointed that out and reminded me that in our state, possession of any amount of marijuana is a felony carrying a mandatory minimum three-year prison sentence. Anyway, several months ago I dragged him to the last physician I will ever drag him to, who put him on a drug I'd never heard of called Neurontin. He'd been taking it for several weeks and apparently all it did was make him feel lousy.

Then, one night, he hears this announcement on TV about a class action suit being brought against the makers of a "blockbuster" drug called Neurontin. So I go on the Web and, what do you know — Parke-Davis is being sued because its sales reps allegedly pushed doctors to prescribe Neurontin for eleven different conditions which it wasn't approved for and had no effect on — headaches being one of them. Also, they had allegedly attempted to conceal the fact that there was a very high incidence of nasty side effects: dizziness, nausea, somnambulance, and — especially in adolescents — suicidal depression. Well, that was it for me. I told my son it was over now — I would never make him go to another physician or make him take another prescription medication ever again. The next day, after calling the doctor and giving him hell, I went and bought my son an ounce of lovely, fragrant marijuana.

— **forty-seven-year-old woman, architect**

Inhaling Gasoline   One of the best descriptions of gasoline sniffing as it actually occurs was published in 1955 by the late A. E. ("Tajar") Hamilton of the Hamilton School in Sheffield, Massachusetts, in his classic account of children at work and play, *Psychology and the Great God Fun*. One day, when the other children had gone on an expedition, Tajar Hamilton reports, he found a boy nicknamed Bullet with a can of gasoline and a gasoline-soaked rag. After a few preliminary questions, Tajar (with Bullet's consent) turned on a recorder and preserved the dialogue for posterity.

TAJAR: Bullet, you said you would come up to the attic and tell me about the gasoline and the bicycles. Will you talk your story into the mike, just as you remember it?

BULLET: Well, I was awful mad when they said I couldn't go on the trip. Sure I picked up the axe when Martha told me not to, but I put it back again. Then she said I couldn't go, and Donnie was going, and when they all went I didn't have anything to do to have fun and I began to get madder and madder all the time. It made me feel kind of sick to be so mad, so I went where they keep the gasoline can and I started to smell it.

TAJAR: What made you want to smell gas, Bullet?

BULLET: Well, when you feel bad, you smell it and it makes you feel kind of hot and kind of drowsy, like you was floating through the air. It makes you feel sort of hot inside and different from the way you were before.

TAJAR: And after you smelled the gas and felt better, what did you do?

BULLET: Then I began to feel mad again and had to do something, so I found a nail. It was an old rusty one, and I got a piece of board to push it with so it wouldn't hurt my hand, and I made holes in all the tires except Donnie's.

TAJAR: Why not in Donnie's?

BULLET: Because they're solid and you can't . . .

TAJAR: And after you had punched all those holes what did you do?

BULLET: Mary hollered to come to dinner, so I went and we had hot dogs at the council ring and then we had some games and then I didn't feel so good, so I went and smelled the gas again.

TAJAR: How long have you liked to smell gas, Bullet?

BULLET: Well, here at camp, ever since about two weeks after I came to the farm. I showed Donnie how to smell it. It makes you feel like you was in fairyland or somewhere else than where you are . . .

TAJAR: Bullet, how come so much gas was spilled on the cellar floor?

BULLET: Oh, I just wanted to get more on my rag. If you have a lot it makes you sort of dream. It gets all dark and you see shooting stars in it, and this time I saw big flies flying in it. They were big and green and had white wings.

TAJAR: And you feel better about yourself and about people after you have one of those dreams?

BULLET: Yep, until I begin to feel bad again, or get mad.

TAJAR: Okay, Bullet, that's all for now. Thank you for being so truthful with me.

— quoted in *Licit and Illicit Drugs*, by Edward M. Brecher and the editors of *Consumer Reports* (1972)

Poppers in the Pool   I was first introduced to amyl nitrite during my senior year in college. The father of one of my friends had a heart condition for which he used the drug. He would amass huge numbers of poppers and give them out to anyone who wanted them. I had read of this drug but had no firsthand experience with it.

My friends and I used to get together on weekends and hang out in a heated pool with a whirlpool bath in the condominium complex where I lived. One cool December evening, after drinking several glasses of wine, we got into the near-scalding, frothing waters of the pool. I was already warm from the alcohol and wondered what it would be like to dilate my arteries all the way. I suggested we try a popper. I broke one and inhaled deeply, filling my lungs with the strong odor.

The effect was immediate. My arms and legs felt like liquid warmth, and at the same time I got a pounding in my head. (We came to call this the "jackhammer effect.") When I exhaled, my vision blurred, with small blue patches filling my field of vision. I then jumped in the nearby unheated swimming pool and got an even brighter visual display. All the effects lasted only a few minutes. I liked them enough to repeat this ritual many times in the course of the evening. In fact, I did it over and over on many evenings.

I never knew about sexual uses of poppers until much later, when a gay friend told me about it. I never got into that. My interest was just in the spectacular rush and sensory fireworks. After a few months of doing poppers in the whirlpool bath, I guess I lost interest in having the same experience over and over. Maybe I just overdid it to the point where it started to get boring. In any case, all that was three years ago, and I haven't used amyl nitrite since.

— **twenty-year-old man, medical student**

In Datura Country   I was on a camping trip with a friend in northern Arizona in remote canyon country. We noticed a lot of datura plants growing around us, some with seed pods. When we ran out of marijuana, I suggested that we try datura. Neither Tom nor I had ever done it.

We each ate about ten seeds and drank a cup of tea made from the leaves. That was just after sunset. We started a small campfire, although it was a warm night, and sat around waiting for something to happen. After about an hour, we both started to feel different. I got restless and walked away from the fire into some big boulders at the base of a cliff.

You have to understand that what I'm going to tell you from this point on is not a clear memory. It's more like trying to put together the pieces of a dream. I have some very vivid pictures in my mind, but they don't all hang together in a logical order, and there are definite holes in my memory.

Anyway, I think I found a comfortable place in the rocks and sort of curled up with my eyes closed. Then I remember seeing bats, a lot of bats and very large ones. They kept flying at me, coming right in close. Their faces were hideous. I thought to myself, "I've never seen bats like that." I wanted to find Tom to see what he made of them, but when I got up, I couldn't tell where I was. It didn't look like Arizona anymore, and Tom was nowhere in sight.

I was in a dark forest or maybe a swamp. It was hot, and the air was thick and hard to breathe. I couldn't tell if it was day or night. I kept getting tangled in these vines and roots and had to fight my way through them to make any progress. Also, there were dark shapes moving in and out of the trees that seemed to follow me, but I couldn't get a good look at them to see what they were. They did not seem friendly. I remember feeling very thirsty, trying to find water, getting more hung up in the undergrowth.

I came to some sort of pool. The water was black and stagnant, and I wasn't sure I should drink it. I scooped some up and put it to my lips. It was warm and thick, not at all refreshing. Then I realized it was blood. That made me think I was going to die. I fell on the ground and started crying. The black shapes got nearer and bigger. I still couldn't see what they were, but I knew they were waiting for me to die so they could devour me. It seemed like an eternity as they closed in.

The next thing I remember is waking up in a burning desert, nothing but sand. I was tied to a stake, left to die of thirst. The sun beat down on me unbearably. I tried to call for help but couldn't make any sound. That also seemed to go on forever.

Then I discovered I was in the rocks just a short distance from our campsite. The sun was up; it must have been ten o'clock. My mouth and throat were completely parched. The light hurt my eyes, and I couldn't focus them. I felt very hung over. Then I remembered eating the datura and was able to sort out some of the weird dreams or whatever they were.

Tom was nowhere in sight. I tried shouting for him, but my throat was so dry I couldn't yell very loud, and drinking water didn't help much. I searched the immediate area and eventually found Tom stumbling around. He had no clothes on and was pretty cut up. He didn't know where he was and couldn't tell me what had happened. I got him cleaned up and made sure he didn't have any serious injuries. He slept off and on for the next few hours, then came to himself, although he was hung over even worse than I was. He had no memory of anything after eating the datura. All he could say was that he thought he'd stick to marijuana from now on.

— **twenty-three-year-old man, ranch hand**

I Ate the Panther Amanita On two occasions I ate the panther mushroom. I was living out in the woods in western Oregon. I once ate *Amanita muscaria* but did not get much effect from it, just a little sick feeling. Word went around that the panther would make you high. Most of my friends were afraid to try the panther. I decided to be the guinea pig. I found a medium-sized specimen, sliced it, and steeped it in hot water and lemon juice. Then I drank the liquid and ate half the mushroom.

About forty minutes later, I was feeling dreamy and relaxed. I lay on my back in the woods and saw images with my eyes closed. There was no sickness and generally no bad effects. The dreamy state lasted about three hours.

That experience encouraged me to experiment further, so a week later I ate twice as much, prepared in the same way. The dreamy state came on faster and was more intense. After an hour, I tried to get up but felt very confused and disoriented. I didn't know whether I was dreaming or awake or what was real. It wasn't scary, just strange.

I crawled out on a big fallen tree over a pond and, while trying to find a good position, fell off. Then I wasn't sure if it had happened or not, so I got back up on the tree and fell off again. I kept having a compulsion to repeat the fall, because I couldn't tell if it had happened or was going to happen. On about the seventh time, I hit my head on some rocks and was bleeding pretty badly. Some people saw me and got scared. I guess I looked bad, although I was unaware of being hurt. They drove me an hour to the nearest emergency hospital. By the time I got there, I thought I had died and gone to heaven. I thought the doctors and nurses were angels and started singing hymns. They did not know what to make of me.

They kept me for a while and made sure I hadn't fractured my skull, then let me go, all patched up. I was coming back to normal when they sent me away, about eight hours after eating the mushroom. My face got all black and blue from the fall, but otherwise I was all right.

I haven't eaten panther *Amanitas* since then. I'm still interested to try again, but I would want to have someone with me to watch out for me, and I think I would take less than that last time.

— **thirty-one-year-old man, unemployed**

Positive Experiences with PCP   I've had very positive experiences with PCP, which, I guess, makes me unusual, since everyone says it's a terrible drug. I used it over a few months about five years ago. It used to come sprayed on dried parsley leaves that were then rolled into very thin joints. From one to three tokes on one of these joints would give me a high lasting four to ten hours. My consciousness would alter within a minute of taking the first toke.

PCP would make me very flexible, allowing me to be active or restful. I could jog farther and longer than normal under its influence, or I could sit still and meditate. I could close my eyes and create inner visions, sometimes seeing colorful, changing, geometric designs, as if I had ingested mushrooms or peyote.

For years, I have suffered lower back pains, supposedly due to the deterioration of cartilage between my lumbar and sacral vertebrae. Whenever I smoked PCP, I felt no pain and, as I've said, could jog comfortably. Even after the drug wore off, I experienced no pain from any athletic activities I performed. A few times, I jogged in six-inch snow, wearing only sneakers and shorts, without getting cold. Even when I got back to the house after such a run, my friends noted that my skin was not at all cold.

My thinking was often imaginative and lucid. And I laughed a lot. I would often laugh so much that people around me, even though they didn't know what I was laughing at (I don't remember now myself) would also start laughing. I remember doubling over and sometimes rolling on the floor in fits of laughter. I loved every second of it.

Finally, there was a strange "psychic" effect of PCP, which I still don't understand. Once in a while, under the influence of the drug, I would feel as though a "ray" or "beam" entered my head through the back; I can't really describe it. When this happened, I would have thoughts or knowledge that I would later find were telepathic or precognitive. I would receive a thought from a friend or realize something would happen in the future. One night, I described to a friend a drug bust that we would be involved in and the aftermath of it in months to follow. It all happened exactly as I predicted.

Maybe these experiences were just cases of heightened intuitive power. My unconscious mind might have had all the information to make these predictions, but it took the drug, or the altered state brought about by the drug, to put the information together and let it come to the surface. I don't know, but that "ray" or "beam" feeling always came first, and when it occurred, I would say to myself or to a friend, kind of nodding my head and rolling my eyes somewhat in jest, "Here we go again." I wondered if I were a psychonaut or just a plain psychic nut. Whatever, it was fun.

My use of angel dust, as I called it, finally got out of hand. I was taking it all the time, and people around me told me I was acting too crazily. So I stopped and haven't used it since. Sometime, I'd like to experiment with it again to explore those physical and mental powers it seems to release in me.

— **thirty-six-year-old man, screenwriter**

Nothing Good About PCP I've tried most drugs and think most have their place. PCP is one of the few I can see nothing good about. I've taken it in pill form a few times, thinking it was pure THC. One time, I was about to give a lecture to a large group of medical doctors. I was using marijuana a lot then and went outside just before the talk to smoke a joint. Someone I didn't know came along and produced a joint. He lit it and handed it to me. I took a deep drag on it and only noticed the taste of PCP after I had the smoke in my lungs. I couldn't believe that anyone would do that to me, but before I could say anything, I was called in to the auditorium to start my lecture.

On the way to the podium, I started rushing on the PCP. I could hardly control my legs or thoughts and could only get words out of my mouth with great difficulty. If I hadn't been experienced with drugs, I would really have lost it. As it was, I don't think anyone really noticed. It probably seemed that I was just talking pretty slowly for the first five minutes; after that, I got myself together and was able to control the drug. I was furious, however, and when I finished, I found the guy that slipped me that loaded joint and told him what I thought of him. I've never seen him since, and I've never taken any PCP since, either.

— **thirty-seven-year-old man, medical doctor**

Ketamine Summer   Soon after I began work in a pharmacology lab, I met a coworker who shared my desire to alter ordinary consciousness by means of drugs. One summer day during our lunch break, he handed me the package insert from a box of ketamine. After reading the precautions warning of possible hallucinations, delirium, and dissociative states, we decided to try it that evening.

We wanted to inject a subanesthetic dose, but neither of us knew how to calculate a "recreational" dose or how to give injections. In retrospect, I believe it was this uncertainty that made our first trip on ketamine one of the best. Robert shot first, injecting the drug into the muscle of his leg. Then I took about twice as much, injecting it into my arm muscle.

Within five minutes of the injection, I came on to the drug. At first, all my organs felt like lead, especially my stomach, and I thought I might have to vomit. These physical sensations quickly gave way to an incredible dreamlike state. I lay down and tried to talk, but my words were garbled, and my mouth felt numb. There also seemed to be a delay between speaking and hearing what I said, so that I kept repeating myself in a vain attempt to "catch up" and hear what I just said.

The brick walls of the room began to vibrate. I had to close my eyes to avoid another round of nausea. With my eyes closed, I entered a new dimension, filled with multicolored triangles rotating clockwise. When I tried to get up and walk, the floor heaved up and down, reminiscent of a boat on a stormy sea. I sat down and felt detached from my physical being, lapsing into a state of semiconsciousness. This lasted for what seemed like hours, but by the time I returned to near-normal reality, only forty-five minutes had passed since the injection.

This first experience inspired Robert and me to repeat our explorations with ketamine. We took it every day for the next two months. It was an interesting time. I haven't used the drug since then.

— **twenty-five-year-old man, laboratory technician**

A Space Odyssey Probably the farthest-out drug-induced experience I've ever had was when a physician friend gave me a shot of ketamine intravenously. Not only did I leave my body, I was rocketed out to somewhere way beyond the solar system. Reduced to a pinpoint of consciousness, I was hurtling through the vast desolation of deep space. Terrifying doesn't begin to describe it, and yet it was very transient. Suddenly, it occurred to me that once upon a time I'd had a body and that I really ought to make an effort to reinhabit it, only I couldn't conceive of how I could accomplish that. Then I realized, much to my relief, that the transformation had, in fact, happened, and I was with my friend back on good old planet Earth again.

— **thirty-five-year-old man, writer**

Addicted to Cough Pills I've had asthma all my life and am allergic to just about everything. Allergic skin rashes and asthma are my biggest problems. I've been in the hospital for the asthma a lot of times, and to control it I have to take a lot of medication, including cortisone and pills for coughing.

As a child, I took a lot of codeine for coughs. For the past ten years, I've been on Hycodan, which I understand contains a narcotic [hydrocodone]. Originally, I took one tablet four times a day; now I take two, four times a day. If I try to cut down the dose, I start coughing and get really congested. Also, I get upset and can't sleep.

If I think about it, I guess I know I'm addicted, but I don't like to face that. I've never had anything to do with drugs, and no one in my family or people I work with would think of me as an addict. Most doctors give me the Hycodan without asking too many questions, but sometimes I've gone to several different ones to get enough prescriptions so that I wouldn't have to worry about running out. I know I should try to stop the Hycodan, but I don't think I can face the day without it. I don't know what I can do.

— **fifty-two-year-old woman, university guidance counselor**

The Wonders of Sudafed I suspect most people take antihistamines just because they have been brainwashed by the pharmaceutical industry. I concluded long ago that I would much rather put up with the symptoms of a cold than endure the depression antihistamines give me.

Two summers ago, I came down with a head cold just as a low pressure system settled over the East Coast. The combination caused one of my ears to close up. After a day or so of constant tugging at my ear, it was becoming sore. I consulted my local pharmacist, who, hearing of my aversion to antihistamines, recommended Sudafed. I had never heard of it.

The Sudafed worked wonders right away, drying up my sinuses and unblocking the congested ear without producing any of the hated side effects of antihistamines. It also really zapped me — better than coffee. In fact, Sudafed is so stimulating that, though I now use it whenever I have a cold, I can't take it too late in the day, or I won't be able to fall asleep that night. I think it's a great drug and am surprised more people don't know about it.

— forty-year-old woman

Testimonials to Smart Drugs My secretary responded so well to piracetam (at doses of only 800 mg) that I decided to give her a small raise so she could afford it. She takes piracetam instead of heading for the coffee machine. Every day she takes it, she is decidedly more alert and intelligent acting, and she smiles more. She is overall a much better employee. She says it wakes up her brain.

I first tried Hydergine six years ago with some fascinating results. During a visit to see my Dad at Christmas, he and I started taking 9 mg per day of Hydergine in the hope it would help to improve our long-term memory. The results were apparent to us both within two days. He was in his forties and could remember events from when he was in his twenties. They were as clear in his mind as if they happened yesterday . . . I was in my early twenties and my memories went back to the childhood years. A unique opportunity had been presented to us to sit down and share in the joys that our life had brought us. What a gift!

During my final year as an undergraduate I decided to change majors from psychology to mathematics. I was also running out of money, and I knew I had to finish in one year and then get a job. I started using a combination of Hydergine, vasopressin, pemoline, and a good vitamin formula with large amounts of choline. This particular combination improved my concentration enormously. I flew through that year, taking a full load of upper-level mathematics courses each semester. Not only did I complete the major in the allotted time, but my grades were better than I was used to. I was getting A's instead of B's. I landed a job in Silicon Valley immediately after graduation. In other words, everything went perfectly according to plan, and I really don't think I could have done it without the smart drugs.

— *Smart Drugs & Nutrients* by Ward Dean, M.D., and John Morgenthaler

Smart Drugs: A Dissenting View   I think my mind is just fine, and I've got a great memory. But I'd heard so much about these smart drugs, I thought I'd give them a try. First, I took Hydergine for a month, a high dose: 20 milligrams a day. It cost a fortune, and do you know what the result was? Nothing. Absolutely nothing. I might as well have been swallowing corn starch.

Next I tried Eldepryl. I got a doctor friend to prescribe it for me and was again floored by the price. This one I tried off and on for three weeks. Nothing.

Finally, I went for the vasopressin nasal spray, using it several times a day for two weeks. This time I did get an effect; it made my nose run like a faucet. I mean, nonstop, day and night. As for the promised jumps in intelligence and ability to concentrate and remember, I don't remember any of them occurring. I think I'll save my money in the future.

— forty-year-old man, dentist

Cotton Poisoning   *Cotton poisoning* is the term used to describe the body's reaction to a particle of fiber, like cotton, or of some other foreign substance that gets injected into the bloodstream. It usually appears in two to four hours after injection and causes muscle cramps, chills, cold sweats, and nausea. After two or three hours of discomfort, it usually passes away, leaving the victim exhausted.

This is my understanding of cotton poisoning after talking to people who have experienced it and after experiencing it myself. My own reaction was different in that it kept recurring. I still don't understand it.

One night, I was with two friends, and we were shooting some drug. I don't remember whether it was Demerol, Dilaudid, or heroin that we were using, but it was something of that nature. We put the drug in a spoon and used steaming hot water to dilute it; then we drew the liquid into a syringe through a piece of cigarette filter. We all used the same needle, and we cleaned it thoroughly between uses with steaming hot water. Everything was done in the normal fashion, and we all got high.

After about two and a half hours, I began to feel cold. I turned off the cooler and put on an extra shirt, and I felt a little better. It didn't take long before I was cold again. I asked my friends if they, too, were cold, but they said they were very warm.

I got colder and colder and broke out in goose bumps. I began to shiver and break out in a sweat. My muscles were very tense from the coldness, and I felt as if I was waiting for a bus in a windy snowstorm without a coat. I was clutching at my chest, shivering, and the muscles in my back and shoulders began to cramp from being so tense. Then I started to sweat very heavily and began vomiting. My head was spinning and throbbing. I didn't know what was going on.

One of my friends said I had cotton poisoning. He said that he had had it before and there was no way of stopping it. It would probably last another hour or two. He went into the bathroom and ran a hot bath for me — that was the only thing that would help, he said. It did help some. I was still cold, but the hot water relieved the backache. I kept sweating and throwing up, though. I don't know how long it took, but I was finally able to get out of the tub and go to bed, completely exhausted.

The next day I was okay, but the day after the whole thing came back, just the same, and I hadn't shot any more drugs, just smoked a lot of pot and drank beer. Over the next few days, I kept having recurrences and they kept getting worse. I thought I was going to die a few times. No one had ever heard of cotton poisoning recurring like that. I finally went to a doctor, but he had never even heard of cotton poisoning, and I had to explain it to him. He was no help at all. Finally, after I got sick every other day for a week, the whole thing went away. I've never had it since.

I've had some bad experiences with drugs. I've had some really bad times with opium in India, including miserable highs and terrible chest pains. I've done hallucinogens that were so strange I once lay down in a bonfire. I've been so wiped out on the combination of morphine and amphetamines that I've lost track of days at a time and regained consciousness in awful situations. Except for my being sent to prison, no drug experience or drug-related experience has been so hard to deal with, so unpleasant, and so painful as my episode of cotton poisoning.

— **twenty-three-year-old man, prisoner**

Panic Reactions As a doctor interested in drug reactions, I've had occasion to treat many cases of drug panic. I worked in an emergency room in San Francisco during the big, early days of pot and acid, and used to see all kinds of people come in thinking they were going crazy or dying. I soon learned that these reactions were more psychological than pharmacological.

One time, a father and mother came in with their teen-age daughter. The girl was a pot smoker and had been pressuring her mother to try it. Finally, the mother agreed, but, since she didn't know how to smoke, the daughter baked up some pot brownies. The mother ate one. An hour later, she was hysterical, thinking she had been poisoned and was losing her mind. Meanwhile, the daughter had eaten three brownies and just felt very high. Before I had a chance to do anything, a staff psychiatrist came down and got caught up in the family hysteria. (The father, who had come home from work early, was the worst of the three, pleading with us to save his wife.) The psychiatrist gave the mother an injection of Thorazine and admitted her to the psychiatric ward. She stayed agitated and panicked for four days. I could have talked her down in an hour, if I had just been able to get her away from her husband and calm her.

The best method I hit upon for dealing with drug panics in the emergency room was to let the patients know I did not consider their problems [to be] serious. When a couple of teen-agers would come in with a stricken friend, I'd just say, "Okay, have a seat and relax. I'll be with you as soon as I can." Then I'd mostly ignore them. When they demanded attention for the crisis, I'd say, "Look, there are people here who really have things wrong with them that I have to deal with. Your friend is just upset, and all he needs is to calm down. So get him to breathe deeply and regularly, and I'll come back as soon as I take care of the real problems in here."

Usually, by the time I'd come back, the victim would be looking better, and the whole group would just want to make a graceful exit from the hospital. Of course, if it's an older person thinking they are dying of a heart attack or something, you should go through the motions of examining them and telling them firmly that their physical health is fine. I never give tranquilizers or sedatives to panic victims, just reassurance and calming vibes. The worst thing you can do is give the impression that you think something is really wrong.

— **forty-year-old man, general practitioner**

Different Tastes in Drugs My husband and I met in college in the late 1960s. We were both involved in antiwar politics and did some experimenting with group living and using drugs, mostly marijuana and psychedelics. I found the experiences interesting but after a while did not want to repeat them frequently. My husband, on the other hand, thought marijuana was the greatest thing he had ever discovered. Smoking it became an important ritual for him.

Over the years, he's continued to smoke it. Once in a while, I join him, but I've come to find I don't like the effect all that much. I can't concentrate well when I'm stoned and sometimes feel mentally scattered and vulnerable. I guess my drug of choice is wine. Two glasses of good wine put me in just the right state after a trying day. John drinks wine, too, but for getting high he prefers marijuana.

In the past few years, our different preferences in drugs have become a problem for us. My not liking marijuana separates me from John's closest friends and weakens our relationship. I don't think married people have to do everything together, but this is something important, and my inability to share John's highs bothers me. Also, I find I resent his smoking friends, since I'm the outsider, the "straight wife," when they are around. Yet I know that if I object, I will just drive him out of the house to get high with them elsewhere.

We try to talk about our problem but have not come up with an answer. I just don't like marijuana and he does. It may seem like a little matter, but when we are having a hard time with each other, it comes to symbolize all of the differences that keep us from sharing fully with each other, and I can see it harming our marriage. I don't know other couples who have this problem.

— **thirty-five-year-old woman**

Different Tastes in Drugs — From Another Perspective After two years of living in different places, my significant other and I were finally moving into a joint domicile, when one day he informed me that he had decided not to smoke pot anymore. I was stunned. Why? I asked. His explanation — that he was starting a new business and had to have his wits about him — was rational and indisputable. Arguing with him would have been futile in any case, but, as it was, what could I say? And yet, I've got to admit that from my point of view, it was very bad news. How would we get out of those awful stuck places we were forever falling into? I consider pot to be a really useful tool, vital, in fact. Besides, I like getting high, and if you get high and the person you're with doesn't, well, you often feel they disapprove, and even when you don't, you just can't connect with them the way you would if they were stoned. What I like about pot is that it lets you detach yourself from your point of view, which is, by definition, limited and subjective; it allows you to be a little less egocentric and a little more imaginative in the way you relate to other people.

Now, I don't blame the breakup of our relationship on my friend's not smoking pot, but I think it was a factor. For a while, I tried getting high for the two of us, but the insights I'd have, which might have sparked a dialogue if he'd had a toke or two, he tended to dismiss as mere dope-induced gibberish. It was evident to me that my smoking pot diminished me in his estimation. Not that he loved me less, but he took me less seriously, and I resented it. Years later, when we finally split up, pot smoking was just one of our many irreconcilable differences, but it was a basic one. Pot can't help people resolve their big conflicts, but it can help with the trivial ones, which, in their aggregate, can really take their toll.

— **forty-six-year-old woman, teacher**

A Mother's Concern Even though my son has a learning disability, which always made things hard for him at school, it never occurred to me while he was growing up that he wouldn't turn out all right in the end. Now, however, I'm not so sure. In the three years since he first became involved with drugs, starting at age fourteen, he has been arrested twice (for bizarre behavior) and hospitalized three times, the last time for a period of more than eight months. Although his severe problems began when he first tried LSD, now even pot can trigger a psychotic episode.

Unlike his friends, and even his younger brother, my son cannot handle drugs. For him, they are simply poisons. He knows this. And yet the social pressure on him to take drugs is often more than he can withstand. Despite his history and my repeated appeals, his friends continue to supply him with drugs, even going so far as to smuggle them into the hospital the last time he was there.

— **forty-five-year-old woman**

The Ecstasy of Love
Where, like a pillow on a bed,
    A Pregnant banke swel'd up, to rest
The violet's reclining head,
    Sat we two, one anothers best.
Our hands were firmely cimented
    With a fast balme, which thence did spring,
Our eye-beames twisted, and did thred
    Our eyes, upon one double string;
So to'entergraft our hands, as yet
    Was all the meanes to make us one,
And pictures in our eyes to get
    Was all our propagation.

As 'twixt two equal Armies, Fate
    Suspends uncertaine victorie,
Our soules, (which to advance their state,
    Were gone out,) hung 'twixt her, and mee.
And whil'st our soules negotiate there,
    Wee like sepulchrall statues lay;
All day, the same our postures were,
    And wee said nothing all the day.
— from "The Extasie" by John Donne (1572–1631)

Addicted to Running   I watched my roommate in college and best friend turn into an addicted runner. Greg took up running in his junior year and quickly got into it big time. I think he didn't have a lot going for him then — no girlfriend, no great interest in school — and running gave him a real sense of purpose and accomplishment. It also got him high. I ran with him a lot at first. To me, running was a lot of effort. I always felt good afterward, but at the time it seemed more like work than fun. But I'd notice that Greg seemed to get into an altered state after about two miles. His whole face would look different, and he'd seem to be flying. He'd tell me he'd get a real buzz on from running, and I'm sure he did. After a while, he started running farther than I cared to: five miles, then seven miles, then ten miles. So I'd turn back early, and he'd keep on.

In his senior year, Greg ran in the Boston Marathon. He trained for it for three months and did really well. He said he just wanted to do it once to see what it would be like. He also said it was the greatest high of his life. So I guess I wasn't surprised when, a few months later, he was training for another marathon. After graduation, he fell into a pattern of running marathons every few months, and it seemed he was always either training for them, running them, or recovering from them. His running seemed compulsive to me and began to drive a wedge between us.

Greg has run fifty- and hundred-mile races since then — impressive achievements, I guess, but he's also injured his knees and back and won't cut down. Sometimes, when we've been on the road together, he's been unable to run because of bad weather or other circumstances, and I find it almost impossible to be with him then. He climbs the walls, just like someone trying to kick a cigarette habit. I think he's become addicted to running as his main high in life and doesn't have a healthy relationship with it. But he has no insight into that and won't listen to me or anyone else who tries to talk to him about it.
— **twenty-six-year-old man, photographer**

Fireworks Turn Me On   I get high from fireworks. I love them and just can't get enough of them. Waiting for the Fourth of July is too hard. I'll drive hundreds of miles to buy fireworks and shoot them off with friends. I guess they're like drugs for me. The good ones are often illegal. They're a little dangerous. And they really deliver.

— **thirty-three-year-old man, engineer**

Speaking in Tongues   I speak in tongues. This other language gives me the words my spirit needs to express itself. It happens on two different kinds of occasions. One occurs when I am depressed, anxious, upset, or feel a great sorrow in my heart and don't really know exactly what is wrong. Speaking releases all that bottled-up tension and depression. I also find myself wanting to speak in tongues when I feel really good. I want to express the tremendous love or peace or wonder I feel but can't find words for.

When I speak in tongues, it is as if a voice from within me is talking. Another part of my being — beyond conscious thought — takes over and lets me express what my inner spirit is feeling in a language all its own. I am totally in the here and now when this happens, not worrying about the past or dreaming about the future. The feeling is similar to what some people get from psychedelic drugs. No other reality exists beyond what I am a part of at that moment.

I received "the gift of tongues" (as the Bible calls it) while I was involved with a Christian commune. This group believes tongues is a gift from the Holy Spirit to permit fellowship with the Father. It means believers have direct access to God.

I was once in a remote wilderness area of British Columbia on a canoe trip. In a marshy area around a lake, our group came across big tracks, perhaps of moose or elk. I suddenly felt thrilled to be among wild animals, where man had not destroyed nature. I looked up to see mountains and sky stretch to infinity. I suddenly realized how beautiful the world I live in can be. Then I started to speak in tongues. As I did, I lost my sense of self-consciousness and with it my feelings of loneliness, isolation, and alienation from the rest of the world. I felt connected to all of life.

Speaking in tongues makes me high. It makes me experience an altered state of consciousness. It lets me glimpse another reality — infinite realities — beyond the scope of my "normal" state of consciousness.

Speaking in tongues resembles meditation. One has to come to it with the proper set and setting, to be in tune. I am sure many Christians who speak in tongues feel the release of an emotional burden or, as in Pentecostal churches, a real high; but to have the total here and now experience, one has to come with a desire for it. Tongues is not magic in itself. The magic is in using tongues to open oneself to powers already within each of us.

— **thirty-year-old woman**

Glossary

Cross-referenced entries are in *italics*.

Abscess: A localized collection of pus surrounded by an inflamed area, often the result of a bacterial infection.

Abstinence: Refraining from using something, such as a drug, by one's own choice. In pharmacology, the term "abstinence syndrome" is equivalent to *withdrawal* syndrome.

Abusers: People who use drugs in ways that threaten their health or impair their social or economic functioning.

Acetic acid: The acid in vinegar.

Acetylcholine: A stimulatory *neurotransmitter* in the *central nervous system*, which also controls muscles and sensory input signals.

Acid: Slang term for LSD (lysergic acid diethylamide).

Acid house: A type of psychedelic music with a strong back beat, often played at nightclubs where people take *ecstasy* and engage in wild dancing. Same as *techno*.

Active principle: The main chemical constituent of a drug plant. Cocaine, for example, is the active principle of coca leaf. Although active principles may be responsible for many of the effects of drug plants, they do not exactly reproduce those effects and in pure form have higher toxicity and potential for abuse.

Acupuncture: An ancient Chinese system of medical treatment that aims to influence energy flow around the body by inserting needles into particular points on the skin.

Acute: Intense and of short duration, as opposed to *chronic*.

ADHD: Attention deficit hyperactivity disorder. Similar to attention deficit disorder, with the addition of excessive activity and disruptive behavior.

Addiction: In reference to drugs, a pattern of consumption marked by compulsive taking of a drug, the need for increasing doses over time to maintain the same effect *(tolerance)*, and the appearance of symptoms when the drug is stopped that disappear when it is reinstated *(withdrawal)*.

Adrenaline: The body's *endogenous* stimulant, a hormone made by the adrenal glands; also known as epinephrine.

Adulteration: The deliberate addition of impurities to a pure substance — for example, the cutting of cocaine with sugars and cheap *local anesthetics* to make it go further on the black market.

Alkali: Any substance that in solution gives a pH of greater than 7.0. Lye (potassium hydroxide or sodium hydroxide), baking soda (sodium bicarbonate), and lime (calcium oxide or calcium hydroxide) are examples of alkalis.

Amnesia: Loss of memory, either partial or total.

Amotivational syndrome: Lack of interest in activities that society considers important, such as school; supposedly associated with heavy marijuana use.

Amys: Slang term for amyl nitrite.

Analgesic: A medication that reduces or eliminates pain.

Androgenic: Having the property of stimulating development of male sex characteristics.

Anemia: A deficiency of red blood cells or hemoglobin, reducing the blood's capacity to carry oxygen.

Angel dust: Slang term for PCP (phencyclidine).

Animal tranquilizer: Slang term for PCP (phencyclidine), because of its use as a veterinary anesthetic.

Antidepressants: Pharmaceutical drugs prescribed for the treatment of persistent and severe *depression*. Fluoxetine (Prozac), sertraline (Zoloft), and paroxetine (Paxil) are examples.

Antihistamines: A large class of *synthetic drugs* used to relieve allergic symptoms.

Antimanics: Drugs used to treat bipolar disorder.

Antipsychotics: Drugs used to treat schizophrenia.

Apathy: Lack of feeling, emotion, or interest in what excites most people.

Asphyxiation: Unconsciousness or death resulting from lack of oxygen.

Asthma: A respiratory disease caused by inflammation and constriction of the bronchial tubes with resultant difficulty in breathing. Wheezing on exhalation is the most characteristic symptom.

Bad trip: An unpleasant experience on a *psychoactive drug*, especially a *hallucinogen*. *Paranoia*, panic, scary *hallucinations*, and *depression* may all occur in a bad trip.

Barbs: Barbiturates, such as secobarbital (Seconal).

Biorhythms: Cyclic changes in biological functions, such as twenty-four-hour cycles of waking and sleeping and secretion of certain hormones, and the monthly menstrual cycle in women.

Black market: The underground distribution system for illegal drugs and other illegal commodities.

Blow: Slang term for cocaine.

Bronchitis: *Inflammation* of the bronchial tubes, producing a painful cough and other breathing difficulties.

Bummer: Slang term for an unpleasant experience on a *psychoactive drug*. Similar to *bad trip*.

Burn-out: A condition of emotional and intellectual impairment supposed to be the result of excessive use of *psychoactive drugs*. Also, a person with this condition.

Bust: An arrest, especially for involvement with illegal drugs. Also used as a verb.

Cacao: *Theobroma cacao,* the source of chocolate, cocoa, and cocoa butter.

Cannabinoid: Any of the chemical compounds that are active principles of marijuana.

Cannabis: Marijuana. Also, the hemp plant, *Cannabis sativa,* and its products.

Cellulose: An indigestible carbohydrate that is the main structural component of all plant tissues and fibers.

Central nervous system: The brain and spinal cord.

Chamomile: A low-growing plant of the daisy family with yellow flowers and a pleasant applelike smell. The dried flowers make a relaxing tea that also alleviates indigestion.

Chemotherapy: The treatment of cancer by giving patients very toxic drugs that kill dividing cells, in the hope that more cancerous cells than normal ones will die.

Chipping: The practice of using *narcotics* such as heroin on an occasional basis without developing true *addiction*.

Chronic: Persisting over time, as opposed to *acute*. As a noun, slang term for marijuana.

Codependence: 1) A relationship in which one person enables or encourages the addictive behavior of another person. 2) An addictive personal relationship.

Coke: Slang term for cocaine. (Others are "blow," "snow," and "powder.")

Coma: Deep and prolonged unconsciousness, usually the result of disease, injury, or poisoning.

Controlled substances: Plants and chemicals listed in the Federal Controlled Substances Act, the law regulating disapproved psychoactive drugs and those approved only for medical use.

Convulsion: An intense episode of muscle contraction, usually caused by abnormal brain function.

Cornea: The transparent outer covering of the eye, overlying the iris, pupil, and lens.

Crack: A smokable, pelletized form of cocaine.

Crank: Methamphetamine.

Crash: To experience *depression, lethargy,* or sleepiness after a drug-induced *high,* especially common after using *stimulants.*

Crude: With reference to drugs, raw or unprocessed.

Crystal, crystal meth: Methamphetamine. In smokable form, also known as *ice* or glass.

Cut: To *adulterate* a drug by adding to it some substance to make it go further. Also, any substance used for this purpose.

Deal: To sell or distribute illegal drugs.

Deliriants: Drugs that cause *delirium.* Datura is an example.

Delirium: A state of mental confusion marked by disorientation and *hallucinations.* Fever and certain drugs are common causes.

Dependence: Inability to separate oneself easily from a substance or activity. See *addiction.*

Depressants: Drugs that reduce the activity of the nervous system. Alcohol, *downers,* and *narcotics* are all depressants.

Depression: Melancholy mood; dejection.

Detoxify: To recover from the action of a toxin on the system. For example, treatment programs exist to help addicts detoxify from opiates — that is, to stop taking the drugs and adjust to being nonusers.

Dilute: Weaker, less concentrated. To make weaker or less concentrated.

Distill: To purify or concentrate a liquid by boiling it and condensing the vapors. The method used to make the strongest forms of alcoholic drinks.

Diuretic: A substance that increases the production and flow of urine.

Dope: 1) Psychoactive drugs in general, especially illegal ones. 2) Specific drugs or types of drugs, usually opiates, *downers,* or marijuana.

Down: 1) No longer under the effect of a *psychoactive drug,* especially a *stimulant* or *hallucinogen,* as in, "If you take *acid* now, you won't be down till after midnight." 2) Depressed, as in, "I'm feeling really down."

Downers: Barbiturates, minor tranquilizers, and related *depressants.*

DTs: Delirium tremens — the most severe form of *withdrawal* from alcohol, marked by agitation, *hallucinations,* and other mental and physical imbalances.

Drug: A substance that in relatively small amounts produces significant changes in the body, mind, or both.

Duster: A PCP-laced *joint* (from *angel dust,* a slang term for PCP).

Ecstasy: Common street name for MDMA.

Ejaculation: In males, the discharge of seminal fluid, usually during orgasm.

Emaciated: Thin and gaunt, as from starvation or illness.

Emphysema: A *chronic* respiratory disease in which lung tissue loses its elasticity and with it the ability to exchange carbon dioxide for oxygen. Patients with emphysema suffer from progressively diminishing breathing capacity and may eventually become bedridden "respiratory cripples."

Endogenous drugs: Drugs produced within the body.

Endorphins: *Endogenous* opiate-like drugs.

Entheogen: Positive term for a psychedelic, meaning "creating God within."

Enzyme: A protein produced by a living organism that catalyzes (speeds up) biochemical reactions. Many digestive enzymes enable the body to process foods, for example.

Estrogen: One of a group of hormones, mostly manufactured by the ovaries in women, responsible for producing female sex characteristics and regulating fertility.

Euphoria: A feeling of great happiness or well-being.

Extract: A preparation of a *crude* substance with water or another solvent to remove and concentrate the active principles.

Fermentation: The process by which yeast converts sugar into alcohol and carbon dioxide.

Fix: Slang term for a dose of a mood-altering drug, especially an intravenous dose of an opiate, as in, "I need a fix." Also used as a verb, as in, "When did you fix last?"

Flashback: A recurrence of symptoms associated with LSD or other *hallucinogens* some time after the actual drug experience.

Freak out: To panic or lose emotional control.

Freebase: A smokable form of cocaine. As a verb, to smoke cocaine in this form.

GABA: Gamma-amino-butyric acid, a simple organic chemical that serves as a *neurotransmitter* in certain brain cells. Its effect is inhibitory and depressing of nervous function.

Gas: Slang term for nitrous oxide.

Gastrointestinal tract: The whole chain of tubular structures from the mouth to the anus concerned with the processing of food.

Gram: A unit of mass and weight in the metric system, defined as one thousandth of a kilogram. (A kilogram is about 2.2 pounds.)

Hallucination: The perception of something that is not there, such as seeing pink elephants or hearing voices that other people cannot hear; also, the failure to perceive objects or events that are perceived by others (negative hallucination). Hallucinations can be symptoms of physical or mental illness, or the result of taking some kinds of *psychoactive* drugs.

Hallucinogens: Drugs that stimulate the nervous system and produce varied changes in perception and mood. Examples are LSD, DMT, mescaline, and *magic mushrooms*. Hallucinogens are also known as psychedelics.

Hash: Slang term for hashish, the concentrated resin of the marijuana plant.

Hash oil: A dark, syrupy liquid obtained by extracting the resin of marijuana with solvents and concentrating it.

Head shops: Stores that sell drug-related products, such as smoking devices, drug literature, and other materials.

Hepatitis: *Inflammation* of the liver, usually because of infection with a virus. Jaundice, weakness, and digestive problems are common symptoms that may last for weeks or months. There is no specific treatment.

High: An altered state of consciousness, marked by *euphoria*, feelings of lightness, self-transcendence, and energy. High states are not necessarily drug related. They may occur spontaneously or in response to various activities that affect mood, perception, and concentration. Also used as an adjective.

Hog: Slang term for PCP (phencyclidine).

Hook up: To obtain a supply of a desired drug. Same as *score*.

Hormone: A chemical substance produced by one organ of the body, such as a gland, and conveyed, usually by the blood, to another organ (or organs), where it exerts a controlling or regulating action. Insulin, a hormone produced by the pancreas, regulates sugar metabolism throughout the body.

Huffing: Slang term for the inhalation of volatile solvents.

Hyperventilation: Abnormally rapid, deep breathing.

Hypothermia: The condition of abnormally low body temperature, usually the result of exposure to cold. Early symptoms are uncontrollable shivering and bizarre changes in consciousness. If not treated, it can progress to coma and death.

Ice: A smokable form of methamphetamine.

Illicit: Illegal.

Immune system: Those organs and tissues of the body concerned with the recognition and destruction of foreign substances, such as invading germs. The immune system includes organs such as the spleen and tonsils, along with the bone marrow and certain white blood cells.

Inert: Without activity.

Inflammation: A characteristic response of the body to irritation, injury, and infection. It consists of swelling, warmth, redness, and pain in the affected part.

Insomnia: Inability to sleep.

Intoxication: The state of being under the influence of a poison or drug, with effects ranging from stimulation and exhilaration to stupefaction and loss of consciousness.

Intramuscular: Within a muscle, such as the injection of a drug into the muscle of an arm or leg.

Intravenous: Within a vein, such as the injection of a drug directly into the bloodstream.

Joint: A marijuana cigarette.

Junk: Slang term for *narcotics*, especially heroin.

Junkie: A heroin addict.

Laughing gas: Slang term for nitrous oxide.

Laxative: A substance that increases activity of the bowels and elimination of wastes.

Lethal dose: The dose of a drug that causes death.

Lethargy: A state of sluggish indifference or unhealthy drowsiness.

Leukemia: A form of cancer marked by uncontrolled multiplication of white blood cells.

Local anesthetic: A substance that blocks transmission of pain by nerves when injected into a part of the body or when applied to mucous membranes. Procaine is a synthetic local anesthetic marketed under the brand name Novocain.

Look-alike drugs: Tablets and capsules made to resemble pharmaceutical *stimulants* and *depressants,* such as amphetamines and Quaalude; sold on the black market or in *head shops.*

Ludes: Tablets of methaqualone (Quaalude).

Magic mushrooms: Mushrooms that contain the natural *hallucinogen* psilocybin.

Mainline: To inject a drug *intravenously.*

Magical thinking: The belief that one can control external events by operations of the mind; an attempt to control sources of fear.

MDMA: Methylene-dioxy-methamphetamine, or *ecstasy.* Also known as E and *X.*

Messed up: Strongly intoxicated on a drug.

Metabolism: All the physical and chemical processes involved in the maintenance of life.

Methadone: A long-acting, synthetic opiate used to treat heroin addiction.

Mickey Finn: Combination of an alcoholic drink and a *downer,* used to drug unsuspecting victims, usually for purposes of robbery, rape, or kidnapping. Also known as knockout drops.

Microgram: One millionth of a *gram.*

Milligram: One thousandth of a *gram.*

Mood drugs: *Psychoactive drugs* in general, especially *stimulants* and *depressants.*

Multiple sclerosis: An incurable disease of the central nervous system marked by progressive degeneration of the insulating sheaths of nerve cells and consequent losses of body functions. The cause is unknown.

Mystic: One who aims for union with the divine by means of deep meditation. Mystics believe in realities other than the one perceived by the ordinary senses.

Narcotics: A class of *depressant* drugs derived from opium or related chemically to compounds in opium. Regular use of narcotics often leads to *addiction.*

Neurochemical: A chemical substance produced by nerves.

Neurotransmitter: A chemical substance produced by nerves and involved in the transmission of information by nerves.

Nystagmus: Rapid, involuntary, jerking movements of the eyes, usually a sign of *intoxication* or disease of the *central nervous system.*

OD: Overdose, used as both a noun and a verb, as in, "Anyone who *shoots* drugs should know how to avoid an OD," and, "The last time I took a *downer* I OD'd on it."

Opiates: Derivatives of the opium poppy or drugs resembling those derivatives.

Oral: By mouth.

Organic: A term from chemistry referring to compounds of carbon.

OTC: Over the counter, referring to drugs sold legally without prescription.

Paranoia: Delusions of persecution or grandeur; unreasoning belief that one is the target of conspiracies and patterns of events aimed at one's destruction or benefit. In common usage, the term is a synonym for extreme fear, especially of other people and situations.

Paraquat: A chemical herbicide used to kill unwanted plants. Government agencies have sprayed it from the air on marijuana fields, especially in Mexico.

Parkinson's disease: A degenerative disease of the *central nervous system* that produces muscular rigidity and tremor (involuntary shaking movements).

Pharmacology: The science of drugs, their preparation, uses, and effects.

Pharmacopeia: The total collection of drugs used in medicine.

Piece: A small glass pipe used for smoking marijuana.

Pineal gland: A tiny, light-sensitive organ in the center of the brain, also called the pineal eye, or "third eye." In reptiles, it controls changes in skin color. In humans, it is a master gland of the endocrine system, probably regulating many *biorhythms*.

Polydrug use: The consumption of more than one drug at the same time.

Pop: To swallow a drug in pill form.

Poppers: Slang term for amyl nitrite.

Pot: Slang term for marijuana. (Others are "grass," "reefer," "weed," and "chronic.")

Potency: In pharmacology, the measure of relative strength of similar drugs. If a lower dose of drug A produces the same effect as a higher dose of drug B, A is said to be more potent than B.

Powder, powder cocaine: Cocaine hydrochloride, usually snorted.

Prostration: Total exhaustion.

Psychedelics: Synonym for *hallucinogens*.

Psychoactive drugs: Drugs that affect the mind, especially mood, thought, or perception.

Psychosis: Loss of ability to distinguish reality as perceived by others from one's own private mental productions. The most serious category of mental illness, it is often marked by *hallucinations*, delusions, and disturbances of mood.

Rave: A type of loud, synthesized dance music, often played in nightclubs where patrons take *ecstasy*.

Reaction time: In psychology, the time interval between the application of a stimulus and the detection of a response. In a simple reaction time test, a subject is asked to press a button as soon as a light flashes.

Receptors: Specialized protein molecules on cell membranes that combine with drugs.

Refined: Processed in order to concentrate or purify. Opposite of *crude*.

Recreational drugs: Any drugs used nonmedically for enjoyment or entertainment.

Reflex: A simple nervous circuit. For example, a tendon reflex is initiated by striking a tendon; this stimulus travels to the spinal cord along a single nerve and quickly produces a response in another nerve that causes a contraction in the muscle.

Resin: A sticky substance of plant origin that is insoluble in water.

Respiratory tract: The breathing apparatus of the body, including the nose, throat, bronchial tubes, lungs, and associated structures.

Rheumatism: *Chronic* aches and pains in muscles, joints, and bones, leading to discomfort and disability.

Rip off: To rob, cheat, or take advantage of, such as in a transaction involving drugs. The noun "rip-off" refers to both the actions themselves and the person who does them.

Roll: To be high on *ecstasy*. Also used for an ecstasy pill.

Roofies: Rohypnol, a benzodiazipine *depressant*.

Rush: A sudden, dramatic change in consciousness and body sensation resulting from taking certain *psychoactive drugs* by inhalation or injection.

Schizophrenia: The commonest form of *psychosis*, chiefly affecting thought. It is of unknown cause and is generally considered incurable. Antipsychotic drugs are the treatment of choice and may allow some schizophrenics to function better.

Score: To obtain a supply of a desired drug.

Sedation: A state of depressed brain function marked by drowsiness, inactivity, and, eventually, sleep.

Sedative-hypnotics: A class of *depressants* that induces restfulness in low doses and sleep in higher doses. Alcohol, barbiturates, and the minor tranquilizers make up this class of drugs.

Semisynthetic drugs: Drugs created by chemists from materials found in nature.

Sensory isolation tank: An oblong, lightproof, soundproof tank partially filled with a strong salt solution maintained at body temperature. A person floating in the tank experiences little outside stimulation and can explore inner states. Used for relaxation and meditation as well as to investigate altered states of consciousness.

Serotonin: One of the brain's main *neurotransmitters*, involved in the regulation of mood.

Set: Expectation, especially unconscious expectation, as a variable determining people's reactions to drugs.

Setting: Environment — physical, social, and cultural — as a variable determining people's reactions to drugs.

Shaman: Priest of the traditional religion of hunter-gatherer peoples of western Asia and the Americas.

Shoot: To inject a drug *intravenously*.

Skin-popping: The practice of injecting drugs, especially heroin, *subcutaneously* rather than into a muscle or vein.

Sleeping pills: Barbiturates and related *sedative-hypnotics.*

Sniff: To inhale the fumes of volatile solvents to produce changes in consciousness.

Snort: To inhale a powdered drug.

Snuff: 1) Finely powdered tobacco, which may be inhaled or placed in the mouth. 2) Any finely powdered drug intended for nasal inhalation. 3) To take a drug in powdered form by nasal inhalation.

Spacy: Detached or disconnected from ordinary reality as a result of using *psychoactive drugs.* (A related term is "spaced out.")

Special K: Slang term for ketamine.

Speed: *Stimulants,* especially amphetamines. (Other slang terms for amphetamines are "crank," "meth," and "crystal.")

Speedball: A combination of a *stimulant* and a *depressant,* especially cocaine and heroin, intended for *intravenous* use.

Spore: A microscopic reproductive cell of lower plants and mushrooms.

Steroids: A large family of drugs related to the adrenal *hormone* cortisone. They include anabolic steroids and corticosteroids.

Stimulants: Drugs that increase the activity of the nervous system, causing wakefulness. Caffeine, cocaine, and amphetamines are examples.

Stoned: 1) Intoxicated on a *psychoactive drug,* especially marijuana. 2) Having the nature of consciousness influenced by marijuana and other drugs, as in "stoned humor."

Street drugs: *Psychoactive drugs* manufactured and sold illegally.

Stupor: A state of reduced sensibility, often the result of excessive use of *depressants.*

Subcutaneous: Under the skin, such as the injection of a drug just under the skin rather than into a muscle or vein.

Subtoxic: Below the toxic dose of a drug.

Sympathetic nervous system: That branch of the involuntary nervous system that prepares the body for fight or flight by speeding up heartbeat and breathing and, at the same time, shutting down digestive functions. Nerves of this system leave the middle segments of the spinal cord to connect to many organs, blood vessels, and glands.

Synthetic drugs: Drugs created by chemists in laboratories, as opposed to *endogenous drugs* or *semisynthetic drugs.*

Taboo: A prohibition excluding something from use or mention, devised by any group for its own protection.

Techno: Type of music associated with *ecstasy.* See *acid house.*

Teetotaler: A person who abstains totally from drinking alcohol.

Testosterone: The principal male sex hormone, manufactured by the testes and responsible for producing male sex characteristics.

THC: Tetrahydrocannabinol, the principal psychoactive component of marijuana.

Therapeutic: Having healing or curative powers.

Tincture: A solution of a substance, especially a drug or herb, in alcohol.

Toke: An inhalation from a cigarette or pipe. Also used as a verb.

Tolerance: In pharmacology, the need for increasing doses of a drug over time to maintain the same effect. Tolerance is an important characteristic of dependence on drugs and is provoked by some drugs more than others, especially by *stimulants* and *depressants*.

Toxic: Poisonous. Harmful, destructive, or deadly.

Trafficking: In drug law, the distribution, sale, exchange, or giving away of significant amounts of prohibited substances; considered a more serious crime than simple possession.

Trip: An experience on a *psychoactive drug*, especially a *hallucinogen*. Also used as a verb.

Underground chemist: A chemist who manufactures *psychoactive drugs* illegally for sale on the black market.

Uppers: *Stimulants.*

Users: 1) People who use *psychoactive drugs.* 2) People who use psychoactive drugs in nonabusive ways, as opposed to *abusers.*

Vaporizer: A glass pipe with an electrical heating element used to consume marijuana by inhalation without combusting it and producing smoke.

Visions: Mental images produced in the imagination, usually seen with the eyes closed; also, the mystical experience of seeing other realities or the supernatural as if with the eyes.

Volatile: Evaporating rapidly at normal temperatures and pressures.

Weed: Slang term for marijuana.

Withdrawal: 1) The process of stopping the use of a drug that has been taken regularly. 2) Any cluster of symptoms that appears when a drug that has been taken regularly is stopped and that disappears when the drug is reinstituted. Also called a withdrawal syndrome.

X: Slang for *ecstasy.*

Zero tolerance: American government policy of going after all users of illegal drugs, no matter how small the amounts involved.

Index

ABOUT THE AUTHOR

Andrew Weil, M.D., is the best-selling author of ten books, including *Spontaneous Healing, Eating Well for Optimum Health, Eight Weeks to Optimum Health,* and, forthcoming, *Healthy Aging.* Dr. Weil has degrees in biology and medicine from Harvard University. He has experienced and studied healers and healing systems around the world and has earned an international reputation as an expert on alternative medicine, mind-body interactions, and medical botany. He is clinical professor of medicine and director of the Program in Integrative Medicine (www.integrativemedicine.arizona.edu) at the University of Arizona in Tucson. Dr. Weil also writes a monthly newsletter, *Self Healing* (www.drweilselfhealing.com) and has a popular Web site, www.drweil.com.

Winifred Rosen is a freelance writer and the author of numerous books for young people. A native of New York City, she now lives on the east end of Long Island, where she writes and does landscape gardening.

NATURAL HEALTH, NATURAL MEDICINE
The Complete Guide to Wellness and Self-Care for Optimum Health

A comprehensive guide to preventative health maintenance and the foundation for Dr. Andrew Weil's work on maintaining optimum health. *Natural Health, Natural Medicine* is the bible of natural medicine, featuring general diet and nutrition information as well as simple recipes, answers to readers' most pressing questions, a catalog of home remedies, invaluable resources, and hundreds of practical tips.
ISBN 0-618-47903-1

HEALTH AND HEALING
The Philosophy of Integrative Medicine and Optimum Health

Dr. Weil's groundbreaking handbook for people who want to understand the strengths and weaknesses of conventional and alternative medicine, *Health and Healing* presents the full spectrum of alternative healing practices, including holistic medicine, homeopathy, osteopathy, chiropractic, and Chinese medicine, and outlines how they differ from conventional approaches. ISBN 0-618-47908-2

FROM CHOCOLATE TO MORPHINE
WITH WINIFRED ROSEN
Everything You Need to Know About Mind-Altering Drugs

The definitive guide to drugs and drug use, now revised and updated to cover drugs made available in the last decade. This enormously popular book is the best and most authoritative resource for unbiased information about how drugs affect the mind and the body. ISBN 0-618-48379-9

THE MARRIAGE OF THE SUN AND MOON
Dispatches from the Frontiers of Consciousness

A collection of essays about Dr. Weil's travels to South America in the early 1970s in search of information on altered states of consciousness, drug use in other cultures, and other matters having to do with the complementarity of mind and body. These experiences laid the foundation of his mission to restore the connection between medicine and nature. ISBN 0-618-47905-8

THE NATURAL MIND
A Revolutionary Approach to the Drug Problem

Dr. Weil's first book and the philosophical basis for all of his resulting beliefs and tenets on health, healing, and the mind. Now completely revised and updated for the twenty-first century, this is essential reading for anyone interested in Dr. Weil's philosophy of integrative medicine and optimum health. ISBN 0-618-46513-8